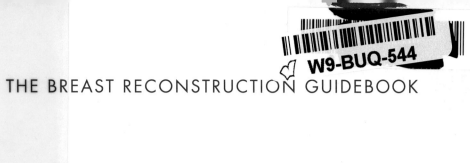

THE BREAST RECONSTRUCTION GUIDEBOOK

KATHY STELIGO

THE BREAST RECONSTRUCTION GUIDEBOOK

Issues and Answers

from Research to Recovery

THIRD EDITION

THE JOHNS HOPKINS UNIVERSITY PRESS

Baltimore

Note to the Reader: This book is not meant to substitute for medical care of people with breast cancer or risk of breast cancer, and treatment should not be based solely on its contents. Instead, treatment must be developed in a dialogue between the individual and his or her physician. This book has been written to help with that dialogue.

All efforts have been made to ensure the accuracy of the information contained in this book as of the date of publication. The author and the publisher expressly disclaim responsibility for any adverse outcomes arising from the use or application of the information contained herein.

The author and publisher have made reasonable efforts to determine that the selection and dosage of drugs and treatments discussed in this text conform to the practices of the general medical community. The medications described do not necessarily have specific approval by the U.S. Food and Drug Administration for the uses for which they are recommended. The reader is urged to check the package insert of each drug for any change in indications and dosage and for warnings and precautions. This is particularly important when the recommended agent is a new and/or infrequently used drug.

© 2012 The Johns Hopkins University Press
All rights reserved. Published 2012
Previous editions © 2005 Kathy Steligo
Printed in the United States of America on acid-free paper
9 8 7 6 5 4 3 2 1

The Johns Hopkins University Press
2715 North Charles Street
Baltimore, Maryland 21218-4363
www.press.jhu.edu

LIBRARY OF CONGRESS
CATALOGING-IN-PUBLICATION DATA

Steligo, Kathy.
  The breast reconstruction guidebook : issues and answers from research to recovery / Kathy Steligo. — 3rd ed.
       p.   cm.
  Includes bibliographical references and index.
  ISBN 978-1-4214-0719-7 (hdbk. : alk. paper) —
  ISBN 978-1-4214-0720-3 (pbk. : alk. paper) —
  ISBN 978-1-4214-0783-8 (electronic) —
  ISBN 1-4214-0719-1 (hdbk. : alk. paper) —
  ISBN 1-4214-0720-5 (pbk. : alk. paper) —
  ISBN 1-4214-0783-3 (electronic)
  1. Mammaplasty—Popular works. 2. Musculo-cutaneous flaps—Popular works. 3. Mammaplasty—Complications—Popular works. 4. Women—Health and hygiene—Popular works. 5. Breast—Cancer—Surgery—Popular works. 6. Breast—Cancer—Patients—Rehabilitation—Popular works. I. Title.
  RD539.8.S73 2013
  618.1'90592—dc23   2012008908

A catalog record for this book is available from the British Library.

Special discounts are available for bulk purchases of this book. For more information, please contact Special Sales at 410-516-6936 or specialsales@press.jhu.edu.

The Johns Hopkins University Press uses environmentally friendly book materials, including recycled text paper that is composed of at least 30 percent post-consumer waste, whenever possible.

Contents

Foreword

Debbie Horwitz
Breast Cancer Survivor
Project Creator, *Myself: Together Again*

I am no stranger to breast cancer. I am a seven-year survivor at age 39, my mom's exact age when she died of this disease. When I was diagnosed, my breast surgeon recommended lumpectomy, saying that getting rid of the tumor in my right breast would cure my cancer as effectively as a mastectomy. But if I chose that option, and also chose to keep my healthy breast, it was what he couldn't remove or cure that would worry me and cause anxiety for the rest of my life. My surgeon wanted me to consider all of the losses from mastectomy. He was concerned that intimacy would be a problem for me after a double mastectomy and that breastfeeding would not be an option. I did consider all of his points—the pros, the cons, and everything in between—when I was making my treatment decisions, but I kept coming back to the idea of doing whatever it would take to never again be diagnosed with this disease. I can't help but wonder: What if I wasn't such a strong advocate for myself at the time of diagnosis? If I had never questioned my surgeon's advice, would I be okay with how things turned out? Would I still be a survivor today?

Deciding to have a double mastectomy is not something I have any regrets about. Taking this more aggressive route may not be right for everyone, but in my heart and my mind, this was my only alternative. I have to be honest and say that I miss the body I used to have. Getting comfortable with my new body was far from an overnight process. Even after the saline implants and nipple tattooing were completed, there were moments when I longed for my old self. The scars never really go away. They fade, but when you look closely at yourself, they are still a reminder that cancer was once there. But I'm still pleased with my reconstruction results and feel thankful that I look close to normal. I've grown into the body that I have now, and no matter how difficult the process was in getting here, it was worth it to feel complete. Reconstruction was the right choice for me. It is not what everyone chooses, and I understand why that is, but for me there are no regrets. Today, in terms of symmetry and my overall look, I know I made a good choice. More important, in terms of my mental health, I think I am in a good place in my life now because I trusted my gut feelings and didn't allow the research to override my instincts.

In this book, Kathy Steligo provides all the information you need to know about reconstruction, including the emotional aspects and the time it takes to adjust to your new breasts and your new self. This is not talked about in much of the literature—the idea that breast reconstruction really is life-changing in so many ways. As a young survivor, I will tell you that I am so fortunate not to have suffered the same fate as my mother. The things I had to give up in my life as a result of losing my breasts were true losses, but they hold no comparison to my feelings of being alive and living a full life.

Kathy, I know I speak for so many women when I say thank you for your accurate description of reconstruction in the pages of this easy-to-read book, and for continuing the conversation about reconstruction that begins in the surgeon's office—the conversation that seems too overwhelming to hear in just one appointment. You are honest, you answer our questions, you ease our fears, and you get us prepared. I have learned that the rest is up to us: listening to our own feelings and trusting ourselves, advocating for what feels right, grieving, accepting our choices, and moving forward and embracing our new self. For me, it's been a continuing process over the seven years since my surgery. I am still sorting it all out, but each day has brought more understanding, more healing, and more happiness.

For all of you taking on breast reconstruction, after you finish the last page of this book, do yourself a favor and keep the topic open. Because reconstruction truly is life-changing, and we are not expected to "get it all" after we close a book. Let this book be your guide, then allow your mind to process and your heart to feel, and know that it is possible to feel whole again.

Wishing you good health and happiness.

Acknowledgments

Sincere thanks to all those who shared their experiences and insights about mastectomy and reconstruction.

My gratitude goes to the busy surgeons who took the time to provide their expert opinions and patients' photos: Drs. Rudolph Buntic, Frank Della-Croce, Gail Lebovic, Joshua Levine, Michel Saint-Cyr, and C. Andrew Salzberg. Thank you also to Amoena USA Corporation, Lori Bruckheim, Amy Burgess, and Tony Cane-Honeysett for contributing photos.

And much appreciation goes to individuals who offered invaluable comments and input: Minas Chrysopoulo, MD; Sue Friedman, DVM; Negin Griffith, MD; Christine Laronga, MD; and Anya Prince.

THE BREAST RECONSTRUCTION GUIDEBOOK

Introduction

Much has changed in the decade since the first edition of *The Breast Reconstruction Guidebook* was written. If you are facing mastectomy to treat or prevent breast cancer, these changes are good news. More surgeons are embracing the concept of breast reconstruction as art. They're using technology and innovation to restore the breast's natural shape and soft contour, shorten the traditional reconstruction timeline, and improve recovery intervals. Your breasts can be rebuilt with implants or with your own tissue—both have benefited from significant enhancements in recent years.

Newer generation FDA-approved saline and silicone implants are expected to rupture less frequently and last longer, and many surgeons now perform single-step, direct-to-implant reconstruction—that means you come out of mastectomy surgery much the way you went in: with full-sized breasts. This type of reconstruction is made possible by nipple-sparing mastectomy, a surgery that was considered experimental and inadvisable just a few years ago but is now an acceptable and available option for many women. It removes breast tissue while preserving your nipple and areola, so your reconstructed breast includes a small but significant part of your original breast.

The increasing availability of natural tissue reconstruction is also encouraging. Your back, hips, thighs, or buttocks can be a source of fatty tissue to re-form your breasts. If you're a woman who carries excess weight in your abdomen, reconstruction provides a double benefit: new breasts *and* a tummy tuck. While all of these tissue procedures use skin and fat for the new breast, some of them also require muscle, and that can mean reduced muscle strength at the donor site. The good news about natural tissue reconstruction is that, increasingly, more surgeons are offering microsurgery, a sophisticated surgical technique that accomplishes the same goal while preserving all muscle. Ten years ago, only a handful of surgeons were qualified to provide this meticulous reconstruction. Now many surgeons in private practice, cancer centers, and university hospitals across the country offer muscle-sparing procedures.

Whether you're facing mastectomy to treat breast cancer or to reduce your hereditary risk of developing the disease, you may be feeling fear, anger, confusion, remorse, anxiety—some or all of these emotions—and you undoubtedly have many questions. What will your body and life be like after such a significant part of you is lost? What alternatives are available to restore and reshape your post-mastectomy body? Will a reconstructed breast look real? What is recovery like, and how long will it be before you're back to your normal activities? Will your reconstructed breasts actually feel a part of you?

In this book, you'll find answers to your questions and many that you probably haven't thought of. Expert surgeons add their perspectives, and women who have been where you are now share their poignant and honest input about the mastectomy and reconstruction experience. You won't find specific recommendations here for one procedure or another, but you will discover an understanding of what to expect from mastectomy and what reconstruction involves. Armed with this objective information, you'll be better prepared to discuss with surgeons the benefits and limitations of various techniques, to decide for yourself whether reconstruction is something you would like to pursue, and to determine which reconstructive method, if any, best matches your personal preferences and priorities.

You'll discover:

- how mastectomy is performed and how it affects reconstruction
- what to expect, whether or not you have breast reconstruction
- the difference between reconstruction with breast implants and with your own tissue
- steps to help you compare alternatives and make the right decision
- how to choose the right plastic surgeon
- tips to help you prepare for surgery, the hospital experience, and recovery
- strategies for dealing with your insurance company, especially if your request for reconstruction is denied

- how to take action if you develop problems or you're unhappy with your results
- information for your family and friends

Maybe you already have a particular procedure in mind, or you're trying to decide between implants and tissue reconstruction. Perhaps you're overwhelmed and just not sure what you should do. This book explains all your options. You may not be a candidate for all of them. If you've undergone radiation for breast cancer, for example, that poses some limitations. Some choices may not interest you, because of the investment in time or recovery. What's most important, particularly if you're feeling that you'll never be the same, is that you can have symmetrical, softly sloped breasts after mastectomy. Reconstruction isn't always easy, and it's not perfect. It cannot undo everything mastectomy takes away or replace lost sensation or the ability to breastfeed. But it can restore your post-mastectomy profile and profoundly affect your self-image and peace of mind.

As someone who has twice confronted breast cancer and twice had reconstruction, I understand just how you feel. I asked the same questions myself. I know firsthand that sorting through the various reconstructive options can be a confusing, time-intensive, and frustrating experience. By the time you've read through this book, you'll feel more confident in your understanding of your post-mastectomy options.

You may decide to go ahead with reconstruction. You may not. Either way, you'll know what to expect. Armed with the right information, you'll be prepared to make decisions that are right for you.

PART ONE ○ DECISION: MASTECTOMY

CHAPTER ONE

Why Mastectomy?

We have two options, medically and emotionally:
give up, or fight like hell.   —LANCE ARMSTRONG

Breast cancer isn't new. It has plagued women throughout history, and for centuries it has been addressed with surgery. Around AD 180, Leonides of Alexandria may have been the first to recommend surgery to remove a breast tumor; having a patient who survived *mastectomy* (breast removal) is credited to Greek physician Galen, a hundred years later.[1] The first documented evidence of mastectomy (without benefit of anesthesia) is believed to be that written in 1811 by novelist Fanny Burney. In a letter to her sister, Burney described how her breast was removed by one of Napoleon's surgeons, after she had been fortified with just a single wine cordial. Although surgery without anesthesia seems unimaginable now, the mastectomy was a success, and Burney lived for another 29 years. Seventy years later, renowned surgeon William Halsted introduced the *radical mastectomy*, with two benefits his predecessors didn't have: anesthesia and sterilization of both the wound and surgical instruments. At the time, the biology of *breast cancer* wasn't understood or advanced sufficiently to address individual condition or tumor size or to provide treatment choices. Breast cancer was recognized as a local disease that was best treated by removing the entire breast and all the tissue surrounding it. Once the cancer was diagnosed, a woman's breast, chest wall muscles, and all underarm lymph nodes were removed, leaving her with a flat or concave chest, arm weakness, lingering pain, and various other complications for the remainder of her life. Halsted's procedure became standard treatment for most women diagnosed with breast cancer, and although it was disfiguring, it saved many women's lives. Absent other effective methods, Halsted's mastectomy became the accepted treatment for breast cancer until the late 1970s, when surgeons discovered that removing only the tumor and breast tissue was as effective for most women and far less debilitating.

Just a generation ago, breast cancers weren't usually diagnosed until the tumors were advanced. Today, a greater understanding of breast cancers, early detection, and sophisticated surgical techniques provide vastly improved options. Surgeons are still key players when breast cancer is diagnosed, but they are participants in multidisciplinary medical teams that assess and coordinate each patient's treatment. Yet despite encouraging advances that find numerous breast cancers at an early stage, when they're easier to treat, we still haven't cracked the cancer code. While we're beginning to understand the nature of certain breast cancers, we still don't know how to prevent or cure all of them. We've learned that breast cancer is not one but many different diseases that must be approached in different ways. That realization has helped experts replace the one-size-fits-all treatment approach with treatment choices that are more focused, more personalized, and more successful. Removing the tumor and following up with radiation therapy effectively addresses most breast cancers and preserves breast tissue. Although most women in the United States survive treatment, 1 in 8 are diagnosed with breast cancer annually, and 40,000 per year lose their lives to this disease. Many more, even those with early-stage disease, lose their breasts because of this dreaded disease or in an effort to prevent it: an estimated 80,000 to 100,000 mastectomies are performed each year in the United States.

Our breasts define much of our physical profile, provide pleasure, and, for many women, feed babies. We're fearful and saddened when cancer (or the threat of it) takes that away. It's heartbreaking to lose a part of us that is so uniquely feminine. As women, we have concerns about losing one or both breasts. Will mastectomy eliminate our cancer? How will we look afterward? Will we ever feel normal again? In most situations, removing breast tissue does eliminate breast cancer. Afterward, talented plastic surgeons using sophisticated techniques can restore breast volume and shape with implants or a woman's own tissue.

Inside the Breast

Breasts are designed to make milk. Positioned over the *pectoralis major* and *pectoralis minor* chest muscles, milk-producing *lobes* (or *lobules*) are connected to thin *ducts* (where most breast cancer begins) that deliver milk to the nipple. The remainder of the breast is primarily fatty tissue (figure 1.1). Breasts contain no muscle—that's why no amount of exercise makes them bigger. In our twenties and thirties, our breasts have more dense glandular tissue than fat. This tissue makes the youthful breast firm. It's also the reason *mammograms* aren't routinely recommended for women under age 40, because dense tissue can hide abnormalities that mammograms may not find. *Magnetic resonance imaging (MRI)* is more sensitive and can better distinguish suspicious areas in dense tissue; it finds more abnormalities, both harmless and harmful. As we age—particularly after menopause— much of our breast tissue is replaced by fat, and our once-firm breasts begin to sag. Though not usually welcomed or desired, aging breast tissue bodes well for early detection, because on a mammogram, fat stands out in contrast to abnormalities.

We all dread the "C" word. But what, exactly, is cancer? It occurs when environmental, lifestyle, or hereditary factors cause cells—in this case, breast cells—to mutate and grow uncontrollably until they form *malignant* (cancerous) tumors. The tumors continue to develop, usually without symptoms, until they grow into a spot that shows up on a mammogram or as a lump that can be felt.

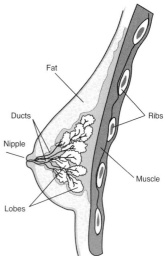

All breast cancers are not alike. *Non-invasive breast cancers* are those that remain in situ, or "in place," within the confines of the lobules or ducts where they begin. *Ductal carcinoma in situ (DCIS)* is the most common non-invasive breast cancer. Too small to be felt, it's an early-stage (stage 0) cancer that is contained within the ducts. Virtually all women treated for DCIS are cured. About 80 per-

FIGURE 1.1. The breast is made of fatty tissue, lobes, and ducts surrounded by skin.

cent of all breast cancers are *invasive*. These are more worrisome, because left untreated, they can spread beyond the breast to other parts of the body and are often more difficult to treat. Most invasive breast cancers grow for about 8 to 10 years before they can be seen by mammography or felt as a lump. *Invasive* or *infiltrating ductal carcinoma (IDC)* is the most common breast cancer. Usually found in women older than age 55, it begins in the ducts and spreads to the breast tissue. Other types of breast cancer may develop, including those that may affect the breast skin, nipple, or *areola* (the darker skin around the nipple). The American Cancer Society (www. cancer.org) has detailed information about different types of breast cancer and how they are treated.

Surgical Treatments

Breast abnormalities are *biopsied* surgically or with a special needle to remove a small sample of tissue or cells that is then examined to determine whether cancer is present. Eighty percent of biopsies prove to be *benign* (non-cancerous). When a biopsy reveals cancerous cells, your medical team will design the best course of treatment based on the type of cancer, how far it has progressed, and other factors. Treatment may include *chemotherapy* or *radiation therapy* to destroy cancer cells, medication to block the hormones that some tumors need to grow, or targeted therapy that restricts or blocks proteins or other substances that certain cancers need to thrive.

No matter what the treatment plan, some type of surgery is always involved when breast cancer is diagnosed. But thankfully, the days of routine radical mastectomy are behind us. We live in an age of patient participation, and, when prudent, procedures that save most of the breast are often effective. Women with a single, small incidence of DCIS or early-stage tumors that haven't spread beyond the breast can choose *lumpectomy*: removal of just the tumor and some of the surrounding tissue, usually followed by radiation treatments to kill any remaining cancerous cells and prevent recurrence. When a larger tumor is involved, a *quadrantectomy*, which removes about a quarter of the breast, may be appropriate. When lumpectomy or quadrantectomy can't effectively eliminate cancer, treatment

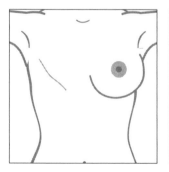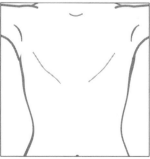

FIGURE 1.2. A unilateral mastectomy leaves one side of the chest flat (*left*). Both sides are flat after a bilateral mastectomy (*right*).

usually involves breast removal. *Unilateral* mastectomy removes one breast; *bilateral* or double mastectomy removes both breasts (figure 1.2).

Depending on the nature of your diagnosis, you may have a choice between lumpectomy with radiation or mastectomy. Mastectomy is usually recommended when:

- cancer is found in multiple areas of your breast
- lumpectomy can't remove all of your cancer
- removing your tumor would eliminate a large portion of your breast
- you've had prior radiation to your breast or chest
- you have lupus or another health condition that precludes radiation
- cancer is diagnosed while you're pregnant (lumpectomy isn't advised before the third trimester, because the accompanying radiation might harm the fetus; it can be performed in the third trimester, if radiation can be delayed until after delivery)
- you have a high risk for breast cancer due to a genetic mutation, a strong family history, or a diagnosis of lobular carcinoma in situ

Other, personal reasons may compel you to choose mastectomy even if you're a candidate for lumpectomy and radiation. You may live too far from a treatment facility, you may be unable to accommodate the schedule of radiation appointments, or you may simply prefer to avoid radiation. Perhaps you have a high risk of developing a recurrence or another new tumor, and after carefully considering your options, you feel that removing your breast will give you greater peace of mind.

The type of mastectomy you have depends on the nature of your breast cancer. A *total* or *simple* mastectomy removes the breast tissue, nipple, and areola. This surgery is commonly used to treat DCIS in two or more areas of the breast or when the cancerous area extends beyond the edges of the biopsy. When women who have high risk for breast cancer choose preventive mastectomy to reduce their risk of developing the disease, a total mastectomy is usually performed. A *modified radical mastectomy* is similar but also removes some or all *lymph nodes* (part of the body's immune system that filters and recycles fluids and removes bacteria and cellular waste materials) and the lining over the chest muscle. The Halsted radical mastectomy is uncommon, unless advanced tumors are found in the chest muscle.

There are absolutely no words to describe the stress and anxiety that unexpectedly creeps up about having mastectomy. I wish I could tell someone, "This is how I feel," but I can't. I feel like anything I say about it, any way I describe it, is inadequate. I love and appreciate each and every person who supports me and cares about me more than anyone will ever know. But this is something that no one would truly understand unless they've been there.   *—Maria*

Finding malignant cells in the underarm lymph nodes (figure 1.3) indicates that cancer has spread beyond the breast and is capable of *metastasizing* (spreading) to other parts of the body. If you have invasive breast cancer, any lymph nodes that look or feel suspicious are removed during your lumpectomy or mastectomy. If your cancer was caught at an early stage and your nodes appear normal, your surgeon will do a *sentinel node biopsy* instead (also called *sentinel node dissection* or *sentinel node mapping*). Cancer cells that spread beyond the breast initially travel to the sentinel node, the one that is closest to the tumor, so typically, when early-stage cancer is found, only this node is removed and examined. Sometimes, one or two other nodes are removed as well. A sentinel node that is clear of cancer cells is great news—the rest of your lymph nodes are also presumed to be clear.

If cancer cells have spread to the sentinel node, it's important to find out whether they've also invaded other lymph nodes and can metastasize. (A positive sentinel node may indicate that chemotherapy or other systemic treatment is needed.) In that case, an *axillary node dissection* will be performed to remove some or all of your underarm lymph nodes. While this is a critical diagnostic step, it often impairs the lymph system's ability to adequately do its job. Fluids may collect in the arm, causing mild to severe *lymphedema*, a condition that causes chronic swelling and numbness. Lymphedema can occur months or even years after nodes are removed. Up to 30 percent of women who have axillary node dissection develop this condition, compared with about 3 percent who have the

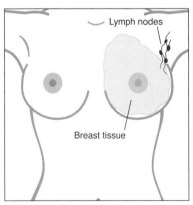

FIGURE 1.3. The body's lymph system includes small underarm nodes that filter impurities from the body.

less invasive sentinel node procedures.[2] Almost half of patients who have radiation therapy after their nodes are removed also experience lymphedema.[3] Axillary node dissection and associated lymphedema may become a thing of the past; some studies have shown that removing lymph nodes, even when the sentinel node is positive, doesn't improve rates of survival or recurrence.[4] More research is needed, and axillary dissection might still be advisable for women whose nodes are palpable (can be felt) or contain breast cancer cells.

Do You Really Need a Mastectomy?

Although breast-conserving surgery is standard-of-care treatment for early breast cancer, mastectomy is more common in the United States than in many other developed nations. American women have mastectomies 34 percent more often than their counterparts in France, for example.[5] Where you live within the United States may make a difference: lumpectomy is more common in the Northeast and Pacific West, while mastectomy occurs more often in the South and parts of the Midwest.[6] Physicians are more likely to recommend breast-conserving lumpectomy in metropolitan areas and locations where radiation facilities are plentiful. Your surgeon's

TABLE 1.1. Comparing lumpectomy and mastectomy

Lumpectomy	Mastectomy
Minimal surgery	More extensive surgery
May affect appearance of your breast	Removes your breast
Outpatient procedure	Usually requires overnight hospital stay
Requires follow-up radiation treatments	May require follow-up radiation treatments
Continued mammograms advised	Mammograms no longer needed*
Sensation retained	Sensation reduced
Doesn't usually require reconstruction	Reconstruction is always an option
Slightly higher chance of recurrence	Same survival rate as lumpectomy and radiation

*If you have one breast removed, routine mammograms are still recommended for your healthy breast.

age and medical training may also influence his or her treatment recommendation. Women who rely more on the opinions of their surgeon, family members, or friends more often choose lumpectomy. When women are more involved in their own decision making, they're more likely to choose mastectomy.[7] Studies show that when given the option, patients often prefer mastectomy because they're worried about their cancer returning or the side effects of radiation, or because a preoperative screening shows additional areas of concern in the breast. (Although survival rates are the same after either treatment, cancer returns slightly more often after lumpectomy and radiation than after mastectomy.)

If you have a choice of lumpectomy or mastectomy, you may be conflicted by the emotional and intellectual factors involved in the decision. Understandably, you'll be anxious to get rid of the source of your cancer—your breasts—and feel safer when you do. It's a difficult decision that is best made by weighing all the advantages and disadvantages of each option. Only you can make that decision, depending on the nature of your breast cancer and your personal circumstances. You may decide that mastectomy is your best option, but before you do, give yourself time to understand all the facts and consider all your options (see table 1.1). Unless you have a very aggressive cancer, taking two or three weeks to get a second opinion will be well worth your time. You have nothing to lose, and it just might save your breast. If you decide mastectomy is your best course of action, you have choices about how you'll look after your breast is removed.

CHAPTER TWO

Mastectomy without Reconstruction

No one can make you feel inferior without your permission.
—**ELEANOR ROOSEVELT**

Years ago, a flat chest was the only alternative after mastectomy. For some women, it's still the option of choice. Even though we seem to hear more about women who choose *breast reconstruction*, others are quite comfortable not replacing their breasts. You might decide against reconstruction if you:

- want the simplest and fastest recovery
- don't consider a flat chest to be a significant change from your natural breasts
- don't want to endure additional surgery and recovery
- fear potential complications or unsatisfactory results with reconstruction
- don't want breasts that have little or no feeling or that aren't "real"
- want to try going flat before committing to reconstructive surgery
- are unsure about reconstruction at the time of your mastectomy
- have a health condition or pending treatment that precludes reconstruction
- prefer to embrace your flat chest as a way of acknowledging your post-cancer persona

What to Expect

The goal of mastectomy is always to remove as much breast tissue as possible, whether or not you have breast reconstruction. If you don't have reconstruction at the time of your mastectomy, a broad elliptical incision is made across your breast, removing the nipple and areola and any previous biopsy scars. The breast tissue, tumor, and most of the skin are then removed, leaving two thin flaps of skin on either side of the incision. These flap edges are pulled together and closed around a surgical drain, which remains in place for a few days to drain fluids away from your chest while you heal (more on drains in chapter 14).

Ideally, your breast surgeon will try to leave your chest surface as smooth as possible. The incision should extend far enough to create a smooth surface without forming *dog ears* (lumps of puckered skin) at the ends. A unilateral mastectomy lasts an hour or so, and an entire bilateral process takes about two to three hours, depending on the nature of your mastectomy. Patients usually spend at least one night in the hospital, although some go home the same day. If post-op problems develop, you might need to stay another night. You'll be up and walking around the next day; however, you'll need extra rest for a few days. A member of your surgeon's staff will demonstrate gentle movements to prevent stiffness in your shoulder and arm. Performing these exercises daily will gradually restore the full range of motion, strength, and mobility in your chest, shoulders, and arm. It may take four to six weeks until you resume all of your normal routine.

Unless complications occur, you may be surprised to feel little or no pain, because nerves are severed when tissue is removed. Your chest will be numb and may feel heavy, and you may feel a pulling sensation under your arm; this continues to improve as your chest heals. Prescribed medication will control any discomfort in the first few days after your surgery, and then you can use over-the-counter medication as you need it. Your chest will be flat or, in some cases, may be slightly concave. Initially, your incision will be red and prominent. It fades noticeably after several months, becoming less visible thereafter, but remains across your chest, even if you have reconstruction later on. As more than one patient has said, mastectomy scars are a reminder that you've lost a breast; they're also a reminder that you've survived. Three informative sources about mastectomy without reconstruction are BreastFree (www.breastfree.org), Flattops (http://flattops.webs.com), and EmbracingMastectomy.com (www.embracingmastectomy.com).

Having a BRCA1 mutation, my risk reduction plan included preventative mastectomies without reconstruction. As a physician and a caregiver for a cancer patient, I wanted to quickly get back to my life. I felt lucky that my lifestyle, personality, and relationships weren't focused on my breasts, and I didn't want to bother with mastectomy bras and prostheses. With no reconstruction to worry about, I had only minor issues with healing, which weren't at all traumatic. But I worried about what people would think about my choice, and how I would cope with prominent scars; they run unevenly across my chest with an inch gap in-between, which isn't the ideal cosmetic appearance. After a year, they faded to my natural skin color. Three years later, I'm proud and pleased to have acted so quickly and adapted so well to this big challenge and major surgery. I've moved forward with my life, and I never worry about how my activities will affect my chest. I'm confident in my ability to do a self exam of my chest and find any future cancer. My scars sometimes attract my attention when I look in the mirror—often I just see me. And no one has ever commented about noticing that I go flat. I wouldn't have done anything differently.   —Margaret

I had an epiphany when I woke up after my mastectomy: I thought I would lose my sex appeal and femininity, but that didn't happen. I spent many years with a knock-out curvaceous body, now I'm okay with the new me and I've never regretted my decision. I found my spirit, my beauty, my confidence . . . myself. I've never worn my breast forms. I go flat and I'm not embarrassed. I look great and I'm still turning heads; most people don't even know I have no breasts. A surprising benefit to having no breasts is that when I hug my husband, we are chest to chest, skin to skin—closer than we ever were before when my breasts were "in the way." It's a nice feeling.   —Sangria

The Prosthesis Alternative

After bilateral mastectomies, you may prefer the comfort of simply being flat, or you may like to wear *prostheses*, breast forms worn under your clothes to give the appearance of natural breasts. Tucked into pockets of specially made bras, lingerie, and swimsuits, prostheses restore your shape and profile. (Partial prostheses are also available to fill out post-lumpectomy indentations in the top, bottom, or side of your breast.) You can also buy sew-in pockets to modify any bra to hold prostheses; if you're handy with a needle and thread, you can modify just about any bra yourself. (The BreastFree website has instructions for knitting, crocheting, or sewing your own prosthesis.) Some prostheses stick to your chest and can be worn without a bra—try one before you buy several, just in case the adhesive irritates your skin.

If both of your breasts are removed, your new "breast" size is limited only by the prostheses you choose; it's not restricted to the size of your natural breasts. Unilateral mastectomy presents a more practical problem. Because one breast is missing, you may feel unbalanced or lopsided and find it difficult to fit into clothes. When you're dressed, one side of your chest will be flat; if you wear a bra, one cup will be empty. You can balance the weight of your remaining breast and regain symmetry with a prosthesis of the same size. It should also be of equal weight, to provide balance and maintain posture. If you're undecided about reconstruction or you're unable to schedule it with your mastectomy, you can use a prosthesis as a temporary breast during the in-between interval.

If you contact Reach to Recovery (www.cancer.org) several weeks before your mastectomy, a volunteer will bring a lightweight starter prosthesis and a mastectomy camisole or bra to the hospital and show you how to use them. When your scar heals sufficiently—generally in about four to six weeks—your surgeon will write a prescription for mastectomy bras and a heavier prosthesis. Be sure to get a prescription, otherwise your insurance may not cover the cost. It's a good idea to be measured by a board-certified fitter for your first weighted prosthesis to ensure it fits properly on your chest and isn't too light or too heavy. Try on different styles to see which ones look and feel the best.

Types of prostheses. Prostheses are available in different shapes (figure 2.1), skin tones, and materials and vary in cost. Inexpensive cotton, foam, and fiberfill prostheses are comfortable and fill a bra; however, they have no natural breast qualities and provide the least shape. Silicone breast forms feel and look the most natural and most closely mimic the weight of a natural breast (the silicone used isn't the same material used in breast implants). You can buy them with or without nipples, and you can buy stick-on nipples for more flexibility. Silicone prostheses are heavier than cotton or foam and can be uncomfortably hot in the summer or when a menopausal hot flash occurs. Lightweight silicone prostheses are also available. Very light breast forms made of thousands of plastic microbeads and covered with soft fabric are another alternative; they're like bean bags with tiny beads that mold to your body.

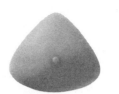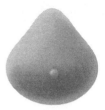

Where to shop. Nordstrom, Sears, Lands' End, JCPenney, and many other department stores sell prostheses in their lingerie departments and catalogs and from their websites. Medical

FIGURE 2.1. A triangular prosthesis fills in missing tissue at the sides and top of the breast (*left*). A teardrop prosthesis extends more to one side (*right*). *Photos courtesy of Amoena USA Corporation.*

supply stores and post-mastectomy boutiques are often listed online or in the phone directory under "Mastectomy Forms and Supplies" or "Prosthetics." The American Cancer Society (ACS) offers a good selection of reasonably priced prostheses and mastectomy products in its TLC catalog (www .tlcdirect.org). You'll also find a wide selection online (try www.amoena .com, www.mastectomyshop.com, and www.nearlyme.org). Several companies will create custom silicone prostheses to your exact specifications. This is expensive and may not be fully covered by insurance; if you'd like to explore the possibility of prostheses made just for you, do an online search for "custom breast prosthesis."

Tips for buying prostheses:

- Let a qualified fitter help you find the right size.
- Take someone with you for a second opinion about how you look wearing different prostheses.
- After unilateral mastectomy, it's important to match the weight and size of your remaining breast.
- Consider prostheses of different weights and fabrics for different activities or occasions.
- If you like to swim, choose a prosthesis that won't be damaged by salt water or chlorine.

Paying for Mastectomy and Prostheses

Although most insurers cover overnight hospital stays for mastectomy, and several state laws protect your right to stay in the hospital for at least 24 or

48 hours after your surgery, some insurance companies still require "drive-through" mastectomies, forcing you to leave the hospital within 24 hours of your operation. The insurance lobby has effectively squashed several attempts since 1996 to pass federal legislation that would mandate longer hospital stays after mastectomy, if needed. With the concern about hospital-acquired infection rates, particularly after surgery, it's advantageous to go home as soon as it's prudent for you to do so. Most women are able to go home the same or next day, but if you need an extra day or two (as determined by you and your physician), you should surely have it. Check with your health insurer to determine your coverage, and confer with your state health department to determine the requirements where you live. Go online to sign a petition supporting proposed federal legislation and keep up with its status (www.mylifetime.com/my-lifetime-commitment /breast-cancer/petition/breast-cancer-petition).

The *Women's Health and Cancer Rights Act (WHCRA)* of 1998 requires insurance companies who pay for mastectomy to also cover prostheses. Most carriers base their coverage on Medicare guidelines, which vary by state (check Medicare rates for your state at www.medicare.gov/coverage). With a doctor's prescription, coverage typically includes one foam prosthesis per removed breast every six months (two after bilateral mastectomy), one silicone prosthesis every two years (two after bilateral mastectomy), and four to six mastectomy bras each year. These guidelines sometimes change, so it's a good idea to check with your insurance company to see what your coverage allows. Many retailers will bill your insurance company directly after you pay a small co-payment. Other vendors may require full payment at the time of purchase; you can then request reimbursement from your insurance company. Medicare will partially reimburse your cost when the retailer submits a claim on your behalf (you'll need to pay the entire amount at the time of purchase).

After unilateral mastectomy, if your remaining breast size changes because you lose or gain weight or due to a medical issue, most health insurers usually cover the cost of a replacement prosthesis. If your prosthesis is damaged (one woman reported that her dog used hers as a chew toy), you should be able to get it replaced, with your doctor's prescription and note of explanation. Review your insurance policy or contact your carrier to verify what your policy allows. If you don't have insurance and can't afford a prosthesis, contact your local and state cancer organizations or the following sources to explore financial assistance:

The American Cancer Society (www.cancer.org)
CancerCare's Linking Arms Program (www.cancercare.org)
Patient Advocate Foundation (www.copays.org)
Y-ME National Breast Cancer Organization (www.y-me.org/programs /wig-prosthesis-bank.php)

Chapter 18 deals with other insurance coverage issues regarding reconstruction.

CHAPTER THREE

Breast Reconstruction Basics

We restore and make whole those parts which nature has given but which fortune has taken away, not so much that they might delight the eye, but that they may buoy up the spirit and help the mind of the afflicted.

—GASPAR TAGLIACOZZI,
"THE FATHER OF PLASTIC SURGERY" (1597)

Someday, we'll control breast cancer. We'll know how to prevent it, outsmart it, or develop treatments that make mastectomy obsolete. Until then, reconstruction is our best antidote to losing a breast. Surgical reconstruction is the process of repairing physical defects caused by injury, trauma, or disease. Using techniques vastly improved in the past decade, talented *plastic surgeons* can rebuild facial features, arms, hands, and feet. They can also create breasts after mastectomy, complete with nipple and areola. Breast reconstruction is more complex and requires more surgical skill than *breast augmentation*, which uses implants to increase the size of healthy breasts.

The goal of breast reconstruction used to be to restore a woman's shape when she was dressed; however, the bar is now much higher: to create soft, natural-looking breasts with gently sloped contours, whether or not you're clothed. This is what good reconstruction does—although some results are better than others, depending on your surgeon, the procedure you choose, and your own physical makeup. You can search the Internet for "before and after breast reconstruction" to see examples of various surgeons' work. The images you find may represent only each surgeon's best results, but they'll give you an idea of what is possible and how results vary.

Despite urban myth and online rumors, breast reconstruction doesn't cause cancer, affect recurrence, or "hide" cancer if it recurs. While reconstruction is imperfect—it can't remove scars, restore sensation, or reestablish your ability to breastfeed—it can soften the harshness of mastectomy and restore your feeling of physical wholeness. (Reconstruction can also help if you were born with Poland's syndrome, a condition characterized by little or no breast tissue; sometimes the chest muscle is also missing or highly underdeveloped—it's like being born with a radical mastectomy.) In the right surgeon's hands, reconstructed breasts are much more than the sum of their parts. They're works of art that are customized to your physique and preference. Small, large, round, high, droopy—we all have different breast shapes and sizes. Good reconstruction can recreate and sometimes even improve natural breasts. Because bilateral reconstruction starts with a "clean slate," some women find that their reconstructed breasts are more symmetrical, with better shape and fewer cosmetic imperfections than their natural breasts.

With your physical *symmetry* restored, you can wear the same clothes you wore before mastectomy, including lingerie, T-shirts, and bathing suits, without special bras or prostheses. More women are satisfied with their reconstruction than not, but results don't always meet expectations and problems can occur.

Sorting through the Options

When it comes to reconstruction, there is no right or wrong answer. There are only personal decisions. For many women, deciding to have reconstruction is a no-brainer; if they're going to lose their breasts, they want to replace them. Others feel strongly otherwise: they don't need or want reconstruction. Many women are conflicted about what they should do. No matter what you ultimately decide, you have choices after mastectomy. It pays to thoroughly research your options and know what to expect before you decide whether breast reconstruction is the right choice for you.

> At 31, I just couldn't deal with having no breasts. If I had to have mastectomy, I wanted to restore my breasts as closely as possible, and that meant reconstruction. —Riley

> Because of my high inherited risk for breast cancer, having bilateral mastectomy was an easy decision and reconstruction was just part of that process. Two cousins had already been through the process—one had

reconstruction, the other didn't. Both seemed happy with their outcomes, which told me there was no right way to go through this decision process; it was an individual choice. Though I had never been fond of my small ugly breasts, I thought I'd be uncomfortable without any reconstruction. Considering all the options, I joked that I was going to the "boob store" to pick out a better pair that was far less likely to kill me. Ordinarily, I would never have considered plastic surgery, so I considered this an opportunity to make me feel better about my body. I had lousy odds for breast cancer, but I was going to at least indulge myself with pretty, more proportionate breasts. I knew reconstruction was the right choice for me.   —Jennifer

Women say they choose reconstruction because it:

- makes them feel whole again
- restores their confidence in their physical appearance
- gives them a sense of control they didn't have with their treatment
- isn't a constant reminder of their mastectomy, unlike a flat chest or prosthesis
- brings a sense of closure to the physical and emotional struggle of breast cancer diagnosis and treatment

It's difficult to pin down just how many breast reconstruction procedures are performed each year, because no single organization tracks that information. However, members of the American Society of Plastic Surgeons (ASPS) reported more than 96,000 procedures in 2011, compared with 62,930 in 2004. The increase can be attributed to several factors:

- mastectomy techniques that preserve most of the breast skin
- increased availability of information about reconstruction
- an increase in the number of bilateral mastectomies performed
- improved reconstructive procedures that produce better results
- the willingness of more women to share their reconstruction experiences and show their results

The reconstruction process. Even though some surgeons offer newer procedures that shorten the overall reconstruction timeline, most still use traditional methods that involve two or more operations over several months. The initial surgery forms the *breast mound*—a breast without a nipple or areola—with implants, your own tissue, or a combination of both (figure 3.1). This first stage is the most complex and involves the most recovery. The second stage, which is usually but not always required, is a *revision surgery* to correct problems or refine aesthetics. If your nipple and areola were removed during mastectomy (as they most often are), they can be recreated during revision surgery or in a separate operation and then later tattooed.

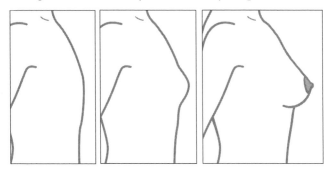

FIGURE 3.1. After mastectomy (*left*), most reconstructive procedures build the breast mound (*center*), then later add the nipple; tattooing of the nipple and areola completes the reconstructive process (*right*).

Reconstruction with *breast implants* is the simplest and least invasive reconstructive surgery. Although the process usually involves multiple stages that extend over several months, it can also be performed in a single

TABLE 3.1. Comparing implant and tissue flap procedures

Aspect of procedure	Expanders/implants	Tissue flaps
Surgery	Two short operations*	Longer initial operation and revision surgery
Hospital stay	1–2 days when combined with mastectomy; overnight if performed anytime after mastectomy	3–5 days whether performed with mastectomy or as a separate surgery
Recreating nipple	Separate procedure	Separate procedure
Scars	At mastectomy site	At mastectomy and donor sites
Modifying opposite breast (after unilateral mastectomy)	May be required to achieve symmetry	Less likely to be needed for symmetry

*Refers to traditional procedures involving tissue expansion.

operation. Usually, temporary implants called *tissue expanders* are placed beneath the chest muscle and slowly inflated with saline over several weeks to stretch the skin and muscle. Then, in a second, shorter operation, the expander is replaced with a full-sized implant. *Tissue flaps* of your own fat, skin, and sometimes muscle can also be used to create breasts after mastectomy. Unlike most implant reconstruction, flaps form full-sized breasts during the initial operation. You go into the operating room with your natural breast and come out with a full-sized breast mound in its place. Compared with implants, tissue flaps are more complex and require greater surgical skill. Although recovery is more intense, the overall reconstruction timeline is shorter (table 3.1).

Timing Your Reconstruction

Your breasts can be rebuilt anytime after your mastectomy: after your mastectomy while you're still in the operating room or anytime down the road.

Immediate reconstruction. *Immediate reconstruction* is performed as soon as your mastectomy is complete, while you're still asleep on the operating table. Your breast surgeon and plastic surgeon will coordinate your surgery date and together decide how your mastectomy incisions can best accommodate your reconstruction. In the operating room, the breast surgeon or *surgical oncologist* performs the mastectomy, and then the plastic surgeon steps in to do the reconstruction (figure 3.2).

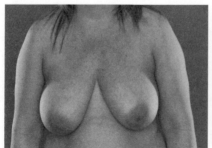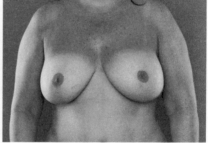

FIGURE 3.2. Immediate reconstruction can replace asymmetrical or droopy natural breasts (*left*) with breasts that are higher and better matched (*right*). *Images provided by Dr. Frank J. DellaCroce and The Center for Restorative Breast Surgery, LLC.*

TABLE 3.2. **Comparing mastectomy with and without reconstruction**

Mastectomy with immediate reconstruction	Mastectomy without reconstruction
Retains most breast skin	Removes most breast skin
May retain nipple and areola	Removes nipple and areola
Two surgeries in one visit to the operating room	Single surgery
Incision is minimized and may be hidden	Incision visibly spans the chest
New breast mound after mastectomy	Flat chest after mastectomy
One or more days of hospital stay	Overnight hospital stay
Extended recovery period	Relatively short recovery period

Immediate reconstruction offers distinct benefits:

- Most of your breast skin is preserved.
- Your mastectomy incision is less obvious and may be completely hidden.
- Your mastectomy and reconstruction are done in a single visit to the operating room.
- You wake up from surgery with a breast mound in place, so you never experience a completely flat chest.

Delayed reconstruction. A postponed or *delayed reconstruction* can be performed as a separate operation, weeks, months, or years after your mastectomy. Oncologists used to recommend that patients postpone reconstruction for up to a year after mastectomy to see whether their cancer would return. Studies confirm, however, that reconstruction doesn't affect recurrence.[1] But a recurrence may affect reconstruction; a breast implant or flap reconstruction may need to be removed to adequately treat a cancer that returns. If you've been diagnosed with breast cancer, it's important to discuss with your medical team your risk of recurrence and how it might affect the timing of your reconstruction. When reconstruction is delayed, the mastectomy procedure is the same as described in chapter 2 (table 3.2)—just enough skin is left to smoothly pull the incision closed

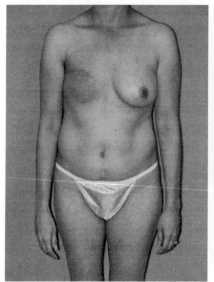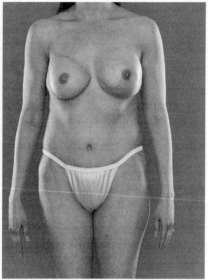

FIGURE 3.3. In delayed reconstruction, the mastectomy scar (*left*) is reopened to accommodate the reconstruction. The scar remains on the new breast after reconstruction (*right*), but fades in time. *Images provided by Dr. Frank J. DellaCroce and The Center for Restorative Breast Surgery, LLC.*

across the chest. If you decide to reconstruct in the future, the procedure will be performed through your mastectomy scar. Your plastic surgeon will reopen it, creating an elliptical opening to accommodate reconstruction to replace missing tissue. The scar will be prominent on your new breast, but it will fade considerably in time (figure 3.3).

It's best to delay reconstruction under certain circumstances:

- You are unsure about reconstruction at the time of your mastectomy.
- You want to try a prosthesis before committing to reconstructive surgery.
- You have a health condition that may add to your surgical risk or impede healing.
- Your doctor advises you to complete radiation or other cancer treatment before reconstruction.

My mastectomy was overwhelming. I just couldn't deal with reconstruction too. I changed my mind three years later when I still couldn't face myself in the mirror and I was uncomfortable being naked around my husband. For me, delaying reconstruction was the right decision. —Copper

My oncologist suggested I wait a few months after my mastectomy to see how I felt about reconstruction. I so feared looking down and seeing only a flat, scarred chest. If I was going to lose my breast, I wanted to replace it as soon as possible. —Diana

Health Matters

Reconstruction isn't particularly dangerous, but like any surgery, there is always the risk of complications. Overall, the more fit you are, the better you'll weather the experience. Though it doesn't guarantee you won't have a problem or two, being fit certainly makes complications less likely. Your age doesn't matter either, as long as you're in good health. Women well into their seventies have had successful reconstruction (even though many physicians don't discuss post-mastectomy options with older women, because they assume women of a certain age aren't interested). Your doctor may advise against reconstructive surgery if you have heart or lung disease or chronic high blood pressure, or your overall health is poor.

Diabetes. If you're a diabetic, but your condition is controlled, you'll require extra monitoring during and after surgery; your insulin or other medications may be adjusted to allow for metabolic changes that occur while you're under anesthesia. Your risk of infection may also be slightly higher than for someone who isn't diabetic. If your diabetes is advanced, your doctor may advise against reconstruction. Your rheumatologist or other health specialist may also advise against reconstruction if you have lupus, scleroderma, or some other autoimmune disease that can weaken your body's ability to fight off infection.

Obesity. Being obese doesn't automatically limit your ability to have either immediate or delayed reconstruction (figure 3.4). In fact, obese women are just as likely to be satisfied with the results of their reconstruction as women who aren't obese, and more satisfied with the way their clothing fits afterward.[2] Obese women, however, are more likely to develop infection, delayed wound healing, clotting complications, and other problems. Surgeons at Memorial Sloan-Kettering Cancer Center found that obese patients were twice as likely as other women to have problems after reconstructive procedures.[3] When researchers at M.D. Anderson Cancer Center compared the health records of more than 3,500 women who had reconstruction, they found that 39 percent of women with a body mass index (BMI) of 35 or higher (table 3.3) had post-reconstruction problems, compared with 31 percent of women with a lower BMI, regardless of the type of reconstruction they had. Almost all women with a BMI above 40 had problems.[4]

Smoking. If you smoke, most surgeons will probably refuse to do a reconstruction procedure until you quit. Smoking compromises your overall health and increases the chances of infection, excessive scarring, and poor healing. Carbon monoxide and nicotine from smoke constrict healthy blood vessels; this is particularly problematic with tissue flap reconstruction, because transplanted living tissue needs a robust blood supply to survive. Smokers are more likely to experience *necrosis*, or tissue death, in the reconstructed breast. This means the skin or tissue dies because it doesn't get enough blood and oxygen. At least one study showed that smokers develop complications twice as frequently as non-smokers and that their

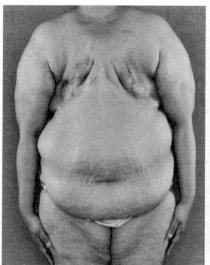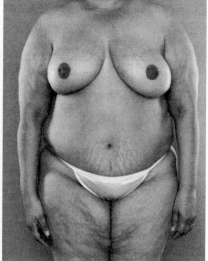

FIGURE 3.4. Breast reconstruction can be successfully performed for obese women, although they may experience more complications from surgery. *Images provided by Dr. Frank J. DellaCroce and The Center for Restorative Breast Surgery, LLC.*

TABLE 3.3. Body mass index (BMI) classifications

Classification of body weight	BMI score[*]
Normal	20–25
Overweight	25–30
Obese	Over 30
Morbidly obese[†]	40 or higher

[*]BMI formula: your weight in pounds × 703 ÷ (your height in inches)[2]. For example, a woman who is 5'6" and weighs 205 pounds has a BMI of 33 (205 × 703 ÷ 4356).
[†]100 pounds or more over ideal body weight.

entire reconstruction fails five times as often.[5] If you hope to have reconstruction, you'll need to stop smoking several weeks before and after your surgery—you don't want to go to the trouble of having reconstruction only to compromise the outcome and potentially lose your new breasts. The good news is that women who stop smoking at least three weeks before their surgery have complication rates that are no greater than those for non-smokers.[6]

Coordinating Reconstruction with Treatment

While breast reconstruction can be a tremendous psychological boost, treating your cancer is always your medical team's first priority. *Neoadjuvant* (before mastectomy) therapy generally doesn't affect the timing of reconstruction. *Adjuvant* (after mastectomy) therapy may delay it.

Reconstruction and chemotherapy. In past years, breast cancer patients who needed adjuvant chemotherapy were typically advised to postpone breast reconstruction until their chemo treatments were completed. This can be a disappointing turn of events when you dread the thought of waking up from your mastectomy without breasts. In fact, research shows that chemo patients who have immediate reconstruction suffer no more complications than those who delay reconstruction.[7] Infection, slow-healing wounds, and other possible complications don't usually delay chemotherapy by more than a week or two. Nevertheless, many physicians prefer to err on the side of caution and still recommend delaying reconstruction until chemotherapy (or radiation) is completed and you've had a chance to rebuild your strength and immune system.

Your oncologist, plastic surgeon, and others on your health care team will determine when your reconstruction can be scheduled, depending on your treatment plan and overall health. Implant reconstruction requires less time than tissue flaps in the operating room, and for almost all women who require adjuvant chemo, an expander can be placed at the time of mastectomy. Chemotherapy can sometimes be delayed for five or six weeks as the expansion process is accelerated and completed. If your doctor prefers to begin your chemotherapy right away, your expander can be inflated during your treatment. If you don't feel up to the expansion process (described in chapter 7), it can be delayed until you complete your chemo regimen. Exchanging the expander for an implant and creating a new nipple must wait until your immune system recovers, usually three to six months after your final chemo session.

I was disappointed when my oncologist said I should delay reconstruction for at least a year after my mastectomy. Intellectually, I knew chemo was more important, but emotionally, I didn't want to be without breasts. I'm glad I waited, because it gave me time to think about my options. —Kandy

Implant reconstruction and radiation. The ideal reconstruction involves skin that hasn't been irradiated; however, that's a luxury not all breast cancer patients have. More women diagnosed with breast cancer, even early-stage disease, are now having radiation. Even though it's an effective cancer killer, radiation changes the molecular structure of tissue, reducing blood flow and elasticity in the skin. Irradiated tissue always has the potential for eventually compromising the cosmetic appearance of the breast, regardless of the type of reconstruction performed.

Asked which reconstruction has the most complications, most surgeons will probably answer without hesitation: "Implant reconstruction after radiation." The combination is not the best, and although some women have satisfactory reconstructive outcomes after radiation, the odds of having problems are quite high (figure 3.5). Irradiated skin can be difficult to

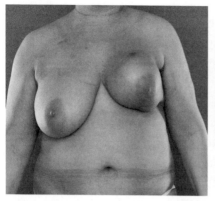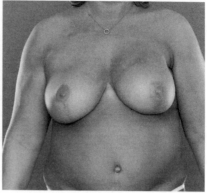

FIGURE 3.5. After radiation therapy, a breast that is reconstructed with an implant can become hard and distorted (*left*). This patient's implant was replaced with a soft tissue flap, and the opposite breast was lifted for better symmetry (*right*). *Images provided by Dr. Frank J. DellaCroce and The Center for Restorative Breast Surgery, LLC.*

expand, and it's more likely to develop infection or heal slowly. Slow, conservative expansion (with a tissue expander) sometimes works; frequently it does not. Expanders and implants produce better results and fewer complications when they're placed before radiation; even then, radiation may sabotage the reconstruction. Adjuvant radiation results in more complications and less satisfactory cosmetic results after immediate implant reconstruction with tissue expanders or implants, compared with breasts rebuilt with your own living tissue.[8]

A breakthrough procedure on the horizon may eliminate implant-after-radiation complications. Three to six months after a small group of mastectomy patients completed radiation therapy, they received two or three *fat grafts* at the mastectomy site with fat that was liposuctioned from their hips, stomach, or thighs (a procedure that is described in chapter 15), followed by reconstruction with breast implants. After 15 months, none of the women had any complications, and all rated their satisfaction with their new breasts as high to very high. Fat grafting appears to reduce radiation-induced complications by surrounding the implant with a bed of healthy tissue. If larger studies with longer follow-up confirm these results, implant reconstruction may become another viable option for women after mastectomy.[9]

Flap reconstruction and radiation. Radiation can also affect the look and shape of a flap reconstruction: the breast might feel harder, have a different skin color, or shrink as tissue contracts. A portion of the flap may die; in rare cases, the entire flap may fail. Because flap procedures bring healthy tissue, skin, and blood to the mastectomy site, they produce better results when they're performed after radiation, rather than before. Several research projects have confirmed this, including a significant study at M.D. Anderson Cancer Center that showed a complication rate of 87.5 percent for women who had immediate tissue flap reconstruction followed by radiation, compared with 8.6 percent for women who delayed similar reconstruction until they completed radiation therapy.[10] Additional research concluded that delaying flap reconstruction for more than a year after radiation produces fewer complications and better outcomes than flap reconstruction within a year of completing radiation.[11] There's another very good reason to delay flap reconstruction when radiation is needed. A flap transplanted to the chest can compromise the effective delivery of radiation.[12] That's because transplanted fat is more dense than breast tissue, and unlike a natural breast, which is flat against the chest wall when you lie down to receive radiation, after flap reconstruction it can be more difficult to adequately radiate the internal mammary nodes and the chest wall without affecting the lungs or heart.

Delayed-immediate reconstruction. If you're having a mastectomy to treat invasive breast cancer, you may also need radiation, depending on the stage of your tumor and lymph node involvement. It would be easier to plan the timing of your reconstruction if you knew whether you'll need radiation before you went into surgery, but sometimes the need for adjuvant radiation isn't clear until post-mastectomy pathology results are available. For this reason, many surgeons advise against immediate reconstruction if it's possible that you'll need radiation treatments. Delaying your reconstruction can be a hard pill to swallow, because it means you'll have a flat chest when you wake up from your mastectomy, you'll miss the cosmetic benefits of immediate reconstruction, and having reconstruction means another surgery and recovery.

Delayed-immediate reconstruction is a unique approach to this issue, one that recognizes the immediate need for radiation therapy and also provides the aesthetic advantages of immediate reconstruction (figure 3.6). As soon as your breast tissue is removed, a tissue expander is placed under

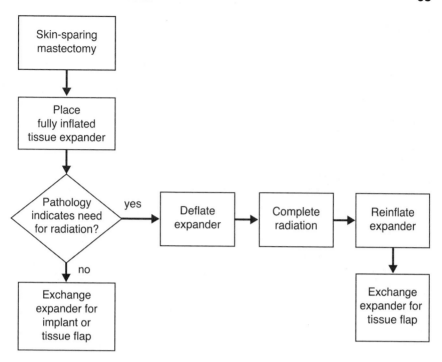

FIGURE 3.6. The process for delayed-immediate reconstruction.

your chest muscle and fully inflated to preserve your breast shape and skin for later reconstruction. If it turns out that you don't need radiation after all, you can proceed with reconstruction, swapping the expander for an implant or a tissue flap. If you do need radiation, the tissue expander can be deflated and left in place, then re-inflated after your final radiation treatment. (Deflating expanders also addresses the concern that immediate reconstruction may interfere with the delivery of radiation.) Several months later, you can proceed with flap reconstruction—implants aren't generally advised, because of the high potential for complications from radiation therapy.

There are no standard guidelines for the timing of reconstruction when radiation is needed, and research hasn't produced enough large, long-term studies with definitive results one way or the other. Some plastic surgeons prefer to "try it and see what happens," while others proceed more conservatively. The truth is that radiation is unpredictable, and results differ from one woman to the next. One day, advanced treatments may destroy

tumors without damaging the surrounding tissue and skin, and reconstruction results will no longer be compromised by the effects of radiation. Until then, newer types of radiation, delivered internally (direct to
the tumor), may cause less damage than more traditional treatments that
deliver beams of high-energy radiation through the entire breast. Mam-
moSite (a balloon of radioactive "seeds" that is placed next to the tumor)
and image-guided intensity-modulated radiation therapy (which delivers
concise, controlled, small beams of radiation to a tumor from many angles,
while "going around" healthy tissues) may minimize skin and tissue damage. Freezing cancer cells also looks promising, but this needs more long-
term study.

Reconstruction and other adjuvant therapies. Tamoxifen, raloxifene,
Arimidex, Femara, and other hormone or anti-estrogen drugs used to treat
breast cancer don't usually affect reconstruction.

CHAPTER FOUR

How Mastectomy Affects Reconstruction

*Oh, my friend, it's not what they take away from you that
counts. It's what you do with what you have left.*

—HUBERT H. HUMPHREY

If you're considering reconstruction, two questions are probably foremost
in your mind: how will your new breast look and how will it feel? Reconstruction is a remarkable procedure. But even the best plastic surgeons can't
replace what mastectomy takes away—your own natural breasts. Although
mastectomy and reconstruction can be performed during one visit to the
operating room, they're two distinct procedures by two different surgeons,
and it's important to understand how one procedure influences the other.

Mastectomy: Cause and Effect

Before your operation, your surgeon will mark the incision lines on your
breast. He (or she) may do this in the office the day before your surgery
or just before you go into the operating room. He'll also mark around any
previous biopsy scars where cancer was found; they'll be *re-excised* during
surgery. This means cutting around the scar and removing it, just in case
any cancerous cells remain. As soon as mastectomy begins, each part of the
procedure affects your breast reconstruction.

Mastectomy action: Once you're asleep on the operating table, the surgeon makes incisions along the markings.

Effect: No single incision is best for all mastectomy patients. The type
and placement of your incision will depend on your breast size (how much
tissue must be removed) and your plastic surgeon's preference to facilitate
your reconstruction. Incisions leave permanent scars. Although your mastectomy scars may be hidden in the *inframammary fold* (the crease under
the breast) or camouflaged later by tattoos, incisions made on the front

of the breast remain there, even after reconstruction. Scars fade in time—most lighten considerably several months after surgery and are barely visible after a year or two.

Mastectomy action: The surgeon removes the breast skin within the incisions, including the nipple and areola. There are exceptions to this practice, as you'll see later in this chapter.

Effect: New nipples can be created, but they will lack sensory nerve endings and won't respond to touch or cold the way natural nipples do. Amputating the nipple rounds the natural conical shape of the breast; if your nipple is removed during mastectomy, your reconstructed breast may have less projection than your natural breast.

> *How Incision Location Affects Breast Projection and Contour*
> MICHEL SAINT-CYR, MD
> Achieving proper breast symmetry, contour, and projection provides the best outcome following reconstruction. Incision location can significantly affect these factors. Unless a nipple-sparing mastectomy is performed, any skin-sparing mastectomy will remove the nipple-areola complex, eliminating skin where it is needed most, at the point of greatest projection. Depending on tumor location, size, and proximity to the skin, additional surrounding skin is often also removed; the more skin removed from the central portion of the breast, the more projection will be lost. In a typical mastectomy, removing the nipple-areola complex leaves an unfilled circle that is then closed with a horizontal, vertical, oblique, or purse string closure. This results in loss of projection; even more so if a significant amount of skin is removed. When a tissue flap is used for reconstruction, additional skin replaces the missing nipple-areola complex and avoids this problem. For tissue expander and implant-based reconstruction where additional skin is not provided, expanding the skin can achieve sufficient projection prior to placing an implant. In certain cases, a vertical closure from the nipple to the inframammary crease is used. This keeps the final incision below the areola and avoids having an incision that runs across the chest. When a vertical incision is used, gravity prevents more flattening of the breast and often provides improved contour with better projection.

Mastectomy action: The surgeon separates the breast tissue from the underlying muscle and overlying skin, removing as much as possible—breast tissue runs from under the collarbone to the bottom of the rib cage, and from the breastbone in the middle of the chest to the underarm.

Effect: Because breast tissue blends with the thin layer of tissue on the undersurface of the skin and is intimately attached to the chest wall, it's not possible to remove all of it, and a few breast cells may be unintentionally left behind. That's why a small risk of recurrence remains after mastectomy. Having positive nodes and a larger tumor increases your chance of having a recurrence; radiation greatly reduces this risk.[1]

Effect: Removing breast tissue also eliminates milk ducts and lobules. Breastfeeding isn't possible after mastectomy, even if your breast and nipple are reconstructed, because you no longer have the mechanism to produce or deliver milk.

Effect: The fine nerves beneath the skin that provide most breast sensation are severed when tissue is removed, so much of the new breast will have little or no sensation. The area of numbness may extend beyond the breast along the ribs and under the arms. Nerves do regenerate; most women retain or recover feeling in the upper, outer, and lower perimeters of their breasts and in between, but the front of the breast typically remains desensitized. If most of your breast skin is preserved, more sensation may return, although this varies widely among mastectomy patients. Nerves regenerate slowly—typically, they grow about an inch per month and may regenerate more slowly after radiation or chemotherapy. Patches of pressure sensation may return after a year or more, but it won't be the same discrete sensitivity to touch, cold, or heat that you're used to before mastectomy. Younger women tend to regain more sensation, as do those who have flap reconstructions, which restore more sensation than implants because nerve endings in the chest often spontaneously connect with those in the flap.[2] Surgically attaching nerves in the flap to an intercostal nerve in the chest can also improve sensation; this is a complicated, unpredictable, and delicate process that requires meticulous skill. Often, it isn't possible, because the recipient nerve in the chest is damaged during mastectomy. The procedure doesn't always succeed, and few surgeons even attempt this.

As nerves regenerate, areas of your breasts may become hypersensitive—it may feel as though you have too much sensation. Although rarely discussed, some women experience *phantom sensations* similar to those experienced by people who lose an arm or a leg. For a while, your brain continues to receive sensations from nerves in the breast, even though the nerves have been severed or removed. As your nerves regrow, you may feel tingling, burning, phantom itching, or other strange sensations in your new breast. These unusual feelings gradually subside.

> *My reconstructed breasts look fabulous but I can't feel a thing except along the outside. Most of my breasts feel as though they've been shot through with Novocain. When I'm sitting down, I can lean forward and not even feel the edge of the table pressing into my new boobs. They could be on fire and I wouldn't know it! You get used to it.*   —*Angel*

Skin-Sparing Procedures

When reconstruction is done immediately, a *skin-sparing mastectomy* is performed. The areola and nipple are removed through a circular or elliptical ("cat's eye") incision; most of your remaining breast skin is preserved to hold and shape the implant or tissue flap that will form your reconstructed breast. Removing the nipple leaves a hole in the breast, through which the entire mastectomy and reconstruction are performed. An additional incision to the side or below the nipple may be needed to remove the breast tissue or reach the lymph nodes (figure 4.1). During implant reconstruction, many surgeons close this hole with purse string sutures—stitches are

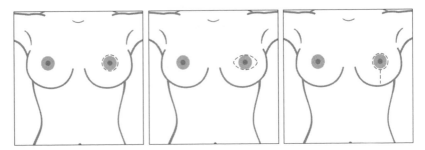

FIGURE 4.1. Skin-sparing mastectomy may be performed through a periareolar incision (*left*) or a cat's eye incision (*center*). An additional vertical or horizontal incision may also be required (*right*).

threaded around the edges of the opening, then pulled closed, similar to a gathering technique in sewing. The puckered scar will be covered by later nipple reconstruction and tattooing. Alternatively, an elliptical incision is closed in a single horizontal line. Some surgeons prefer to fill the hole with a small graft of skin taken from the stomach, thigh, or hip. If you have reconstruction with your own tissue, a portion of the flap skin will fill the hole.

A skin-sparing mastectomy combined with immediate reconstruction produces a new breast with minimal scarring, and later tattooing of the areola covers the scar. From an aesthetic perspective, if you begin mastectomy and immediate reconstruction without visible scarring, you have a good chance of emerging in much the same way. Skin-sparing mastectomies aren't recommended if you have inflammatory breast cancer or a tumor in your breast skin.

Saving Your Nipple and Areola

Nipple-sparing mastectomy (NSM) represents the evolution of breast removal procedures: from Halsted's radical mastectomy that took the entire breast, chest muscles, and lymph nodes, to skin-sparing mastectomy procedures that remove only the tumor and breast tissue and preserve the nipple, areola, and most breast skin. NSM is more technically demanding than other mastectomy procedures. If you're interested in NSM, thoroughly discuss the advantages and disadvantages with a plastic surgeon who is experienced with this procedure.

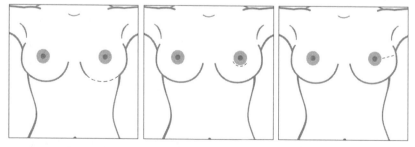

FIGURE 4.2. Surgeons use a variety of nipple-sparing incisions.

Incision placement is critical to a successful NSM. It must allow for removing the tumor and still remove the breast tissue—the same amount of tissue must be removed through a smaller incision—while saving the skin for reconstruction and preserving the blood supply to the nipple (figure 4.2). The surgeon must separate tiny blood vessels that support the nipple from the tissue that is to be removed. The nipple survives if it receives enough blood from the skin around it; the odds of that happening are better when the mastectomy incision is made under the breast or along the outer contour, rather than around the nipple. Other factors, including whether you smoke or have circulatory problems, may also influence the survival of the nipple. If necrosis occurs, a portion of the nipple may die. If the entire nipple dies, it must then be removed and a new one (if desired) recreated.

During the mastectomy, the nipple and areola remain attached to the breast. The underlying tissue at the base of the nipple is removed, and a sample is sent to be examined by a *pathologist*. If cancerous cells are found, the nipple is also removed. (NSM isn't the same as the *subcutaneous* mastectomies performed in the 1970s that intentionally left behind breast tissue—and sometimes hidden cancers—to provide an adequate blood supply to the nipple.) Some surgeons core the interior of the nipple, which usually flattens it, and replace the nipple "stuffing" with a bit of rib cartilage or a synthetic surgical material. Not all surgeons do this, so it's worth asking about how your nipple-sparing procedure will be performed. An argument can be made for leaving the nipple tissue intact, as long as breast tissue at the base of the nipple is removed and found to be cancer free. Some experts believe this slightly raises the risk for future cancer, but there's good evidence to show that the type of ductal-lobular structure where cancer typically develops isn't usually found in the nipple. Cancer rarely, if ever, develops there, so if the tissue at the base of the nipple is clear of cancerous cells, leaving the rest of the nipple tissue intact appears to be safe.[3]

You have increased risk for losing your nipple after NSM if you're a smoker or if your breast was previously irradiated. Although no long-term studies of recurrence rates after NSM are available yet, and medical experts haven't reached consensus on selection criteria or procedure, short-term follow-up shows that NSM is safe for carefully selected candidates,[4] including the following:

- women with only a single tumor that is no larger than 3 cm (some surgeons consider NSM to be safe when there are multiple tumors, as long as they're a satisfactory distance from the nipple)
- women with tumors that aren't in the skin and are at least 2 cm—about an inch—from the nipple[5]
- women who choose preventive mastectomy to reduce their risk of developing breast cancer

Will your nipples be the same after nipple-sparing mastectomy? Many women consider their nipples to be the focal point of their breasts, and keeping them intact preserves a much-appreciated, small part of their natural breasts. NSM combined with immediate reconstruction often produces superior cosmetic results (as you'll see in chapter 6). In fact, it may be difficult to see that your new breasts are not the ones you were born with. NSM is not without challenges, however. Having nipple-sparing mastectomy doesn't guarantee that your nipples will look or react the same as they did before. They may flatten, have little or no sensation, or not respond to touch or cold. If your reconstructed breast isn't the same size or shape as your natural breast, retained nipples may not be centered or where you want them. After unilateral mastectomy, the nipple on your reconstructed breast may not line up exactly with its counterpart on your opposite breast. Before your reconstruction, ask your surgeon how he'll approach these issues and what you can realistically expect.

You'll want to know how your nipple will react after reconstruction—that's difficult to predict, but it's safe to say that some level of sensation will be lost. It's also impossible to predict the degree of decreased sensation or loss of feeling that will occur. Most nipple sensation originates from the fourth intercostal nerve branch that extends from the chest wall—a nerve that is frequently damaged or severed during mastectomy, significantly reducing or eliminating sensation. The fine nerves and small muscle fibers that make a healthy nipple harden and contract are also cut when breast tissue is removed, so even if you retain your own nipples, they probably won't react to cold or sexual stimulation the way they did before surgery—two characteristics you may hope to retain but may not.

A small subset of women report having almost full pre-mastectomy sensation after reconstruction. You have to wonder about that. Did their breast surgeon leave more tissue (and risk of recurrence) behind? Do these women have especially resilient nerves? It's hard to tell. Sensation is difficult to qualify and quantify, because women retain or regain it to differing degrees, and not everyone perceives or defines it in the same way. Assessing the amount and quality of sensation is highly subjective and is usually self-reported by patients. No objective large-scale, well-documented research citing patient satisfaction after NSM has been published. The most comprehensive study so far was conducted by well-respected reconstructive surgeons in Italy, who found that among 773 women who had nipple-sparing mastectomies, only 30 percent recovered some level of sensitivity after several months.[6] Even though nipple sensation and response are diminished after NSM, women often say it's a comfort to retain their own nipples. Others admit they wouldn't have chosen NSM if they knew in advance that their nipples wouldn't be the same.

Even though NSM isn't the standard of care, it's moved beyond the realm of experimental surgery and is now more commonly performed. Not all physicians are on board with the concept, however, and many still prefer traditional remove-the-nipple procedures. It may be difficult to find a breast surgeon or surgical oncologist who has experience with NSM. So, you have a decision to make. Would you rather have reconstructed, well-placed nipples with no sensation or your own nipples that may have little or no feeling or erectile function?

Questions for your breast surgeon before nipple-sparing mastectomy:

- How many NSM procedures have you done?
- Where will my incisions be and how do they affect nipple reaction and sensation?
- Do you remove the nipple or keep it attached during mastectomy?
- Will you check my nipple for cancer or abnormal cells during surgery?
- Will my nipple be flat after mastectomy?
- How much sensation and reaction can I expect to retain?
- What complications might occur and how will you address them?

I decided on a nipple-sparing mastectomy with immediate reconstruction because my breasts were important to my sexuality and I was very concerned about losing erogenous sensation. I knew no procedure could guarantee my sensation would return, but I wanted the highest possibility. So when choosing my reconstruction, I searched until I found a surgeon who would also do nerve reconnection, despite the fact that it is controversial. It took a year and a half, but my right breast now has nearly normal sensation and the nipple has some erogenous sensation. It's not as pleasurable as before, but it is thrilling to have some of the feeling back. My left breast has almost full sensation in the skin; although my nipple senses touch and temperature, it has no erogenous response. I know many women regain feeling without the added two-hour surgery I had to reconnect nerves, so it's hard to know if my sensation would have returned anyway. I feel lucky and just like the same old me, which was all I really wanted.

—Lisa

I decided not to keep my nipples, because I inherited a very nasty family mutation and my father developed breast cancer very near his nipple. I just told the doctor to "take everything." At 51 years old, I still had a pretty good intimate life with my husband, and I was not going to sacrifice my life for those nipples.

—Debra

Right after my nipple-sparing surgery my breasts were bruised and dented, with the nipples pointing in opposite directions. Week by week the bruising disappeared and the nipples evened out. After a few months I was very pleased with my results, and within six months I was thrilled. It took about a year for my breasts to settle permanently. Now the scars under my breasts have faded to practically nothing. I went from an A-cup to a small C-cup, my projection looks natural, and I can go braless without a problem. It was so important to me to come out of surgery looking essentially the same, and that is what keeping my own nipples did for me. My new breasts look like my own and are fantastic! In fact, I'm happier with my breasts now than I was before surgery. I do not have any sensation on or around my nipples; however, I went into surgery well aware of this probability and I accept it as part of the tradeoff to vastly reduce my breast cancer risk. I would make the same decision, with the same surgeons, in a heartbeat.

—Andrea

Nipple banking. Removing and freezing the nipple for later reconstruction was tried many years ago for women who couldn't have immediate

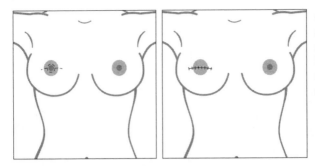

FIGURE 4.3. An areola-sparing mastectomy removes the nipple and breast tissue through an incision made across the areola.

reconstruction. Although it's still practiced in countries where nipple-sparing mastectomy isn't offered, it's considered to be risky—if the nipple contains any hidden cancer cells, they'll be transplanted onto the newly reconstructed breast. Cryopreservation is also unpredictable and often distorts or damages nipple tissue.

A similar, safer procedure can be performed for women who prefer NSM with immediate reconstruction and have very large or sagging breasts. Because their natural nipples wouldn't be properly centered on their newly reconstructed, smaller and higher breasts, the nipples are removed during mastectomy and banked in the groin for several months, until the breast mounds have healed (as long as a pathologist determines that the nipples contain no cancerous cells; otherwise, they need to be removed). The nipples are then transplanted onto the new breasts. Nipples reapplied to the breasts in this way may be flat and have little or no sensation.

Areola-sparing mastectomy. Keeping your nipples isn't advised if you have a high risk for recurrence, but you may be able to keep your areolae, if that's important to you. Unlike nipples, which contain breast tissue, areolae contain only skin cells. In an *areola-sparing mastectomy*, your breast tissue and nipple are removed with a horizontal incision across the areola (figure 4.3). A new nipple can be made later from the areola skin. Short-term studies show this procedure has few complications and doesn't significantly increase the odds of recurrence.

CHAPTER FIVE

Considering Prophylactic Mastectomy

I make the most of all that comes and the least of all that goes.

—SARA TEASDALE, AMERICAN POET

Ironically, in some ways we've come full circle with regard to mastectomy. In an era of early detection and breast conservation, more *previvors*—women who inherit a high risk for breast cancer but haven't been diagnosed with the disease—are choosing to remove their healthy breasts. If you're a previvor, *prophylactic bilateral mastectomy (PBM)* is the most effective way to reduce your risk of breast cancer. Some experts argue that many women who remove their breasts do so needlessly, since not all of them would ever develop breast cancer. Clinically, that may be an understandable position. You might not have the same point of view, though, if you're extraordinarily prone to developing breast cancer or you've seen loved ones struggle with a cancer diagnosis and treatment, and you would like to do just about anything to avoid that fate.

Although scientists haven't found all the reasons that breast cancer runs in some families, the discovery of the *BReast CAncer1 (BRCA1)* and the *BReast CAncer2 (BRCA2)* genes gave unprecedented insight into the biology of *hereditary breast cancer*. While we often hear people decide to be tested to see whether they have the "breast cancer gene," this is a misnomer, since we all have both BRCA genes. Healthy BRCA genes produce proteins that repair cell damage and suppress tumor growth. Most breast cancers are caused by *genetic mutations* that are acquired from lifestyle behaviors or environmental triggers as we age. When these abnormalities develop in BRCA genes, the genes can no longer function in their protective role, and the risk for developing breast and ovarian cancers increases significantly. Only 5 to 10 percent of breast cancers are thought to be hereditary; about half of these are caused by inherited mutations in BRCA1 or BRCA2, which can be passed from one generation to the next. (Other, as yet unidentified genes may also affect risk.) Either parent may pass on a BRCA mutation to their children.

Should You Have Genetic Testing?

Media reports often highlight how a small sample of an individual's blood can be used to trace ancestry, identify DNA in crime scene evidence, and determine genetic predisposition to disease. You might wonder whether you, too, should be tested for a genetic predisposition. *Genetic testing* is the only way to tell whether you've inherited a mutation that makes you prone to breast cancer. But testing isn't right for everyone, and not all families with breast cancer test positive for a BRCA mutation. Most, in fact, have negative results.

If you're concerned that the cancer in your family is inherited and you're considering genetic testing to see whether you carry a mutation, it's always a good idea to first consult with a health professional who is trained in genetic counseling. According to Facing Our Risk of Cancer Empowered (FORCE), a nonprofit education and support group for people with hereditary breast and ovarian cancers, genetic counseling may be warranted if you or any of your blood relatives have been diagnosed with:

- breast cancer at age 50 or younger
- breast cancer in both breasts at any age
- both breast cancer and ovarian cancer
- male breast cancer
- ovarian or fallopian tube cancer at any age
- cancer of the breast, ovary, fallopian tube, prostate, or pancreas, or melanoma in more than one relative on the same side of the family

Consulting with a specially trained *genetic counselor* is an important first step. Using your personal and family medical history, she'll determine whether your family has a pattern of hereditary cancer, explain the benefits and limitations of genetic testing, and determine whether testing is appropriate for you or other family members. If you decide to be tested, your counselor will help you understand the implications of either a positive or a negative result. If you test positive for a genetic mutation, she'll explain different risk management actions and how they can reduce your risk. If your oncologist, surgeon, or other physician offers genetic testing but isn't trained to provide genetic counseling, ask for a referral to a qualified genetic counselor or genetics expert. Or check online to find a counselor by visiting the National Society of Genetic Counselors' website (www.nsgc.org) or using the National Cancer Institute's online directory (www.cancer.gov /cancertopics/genetics/directory). If no genetics experts are nearby or convenient, you can consult Informed Medical Decisions (www.informeddna .com), which provides genetic counseling by telephone.

How Real Is Your Risk?

To say breast cancer risk is a complex subject is a gross understatement. While researchers continue to make great strides in understanding the disease, much about it remains an enigma. The science of risk assessment is far from perfect, and too many unknowns prevent genetics experts from predicting who will or won't get breast cancer or accurately pinpointing an individual's exact level of risk.

For the average woman in the United States, breast cancer risk is based on the rate of diagnosis among the entire population; hence the familiar 1-in-8 statistic. Calculating risk for someone who has a BRCA mutation is not as simple. For this, experts use estimates based on studies of breast cancer rates among high-risk families. Because these studies have shown very different levels of risk, a high-risk individual's probability of developing breast cancer is typically expressed as a range of estimated risk. Your own risk assessment is adjusted for the type of mutation you have and for the risk factors that you can control (smoking, using birth control pills, breastfeeding, and others) and those you cannot (race, gender, age, family history, and others).

Regardless of the imprecise nature of risk assessment, experts agree on one premise: if you have a BRCA mutation, your risk for developing breast cancer throughout your lifetime is exceptionally higher than the risk for other women: as high as 86 percent, compared with just 12.5 percent for women who don't have a mutation.[1] If you have a strong family history and test negative for a BRCA mutation, your risk is thought to be greater than that for a woman in the general population, but less than the risk for someone who has a BRCA gene mutation. Having a BRCA mutation or a strong family history of the disease doesn't guarantee that you'll one day be diagnosed with cancer, even though it greatly increases that likelihood. If you are a woman with a BRCA gene mutation, you have a higher-than-average risk for:

- developing breast cancer
- diagnosis at a younger age
- breast cancer in both breasts
- other cancers, including ovarian cancer, pancreatic cancer, and melanoma

Men with BRCA mutations have increased risk for cancers of the breast, prostate, and pancreas. Having a BRCA2 mutation also raises a man's risk for melanoma.

Understanding high cancer risk can be perplexing, and confronting it is frightening—both actions are critically important opportunities to do something about it. Perhaps someday scientists will discover ways to repair defective genes. Until that time, if you're predisposed to developing breast cancer, you have options to manage your high risk. Increasing surveillance with more frequent breast exams, mammograms, and other screenings doesn't reduce your risk of developing cancer but may help detect any future breast cancer at an early, treatable stage. Taking tamoxifen, raloxifene, or other similar medication is one way to eliminate part of your risk. (If you're at high risk, you'll want to have increased surveillance even if you choose to take a risk-lowering medication.) There is another, more extreme and more effective alternative: preventive mastectomy of both healthy breasts.

Removing Your Breasts to Reduce Your Risk

The most effective method of reducing a high risk for breast cancer is prophylactic bilateral mastectomy, which lowers your odds by 90 percent or more.[2] (A small risk remains because it's impossible to remove every bit of breast tissue and every breast cell.) If your estimated risk for breast cancer is 80 percent, it will be 8 percent or less after PBM, lower than the risk for

TABLE 5.1. Reducing breast cancer risk with preventive surgery

Procedure(s)	Estimated risk reduction (%)
Bilateral preventive mastectomy	90[*]
Bilateral salpingo-oophorectomy (before natural menopause)	50
Both surgeries	95

[*]For women with intact ovaries.

women of average risk. If you have a BRCA mutation, experts also recommend preventive *bilateral salpingo-oophorectomy (BSO)*—removal of both ovaries—between ages 35 and 40 or when you complete childbearing. BSO reduces ovarian cancer risk by 80 percent or more and also lowers your breast cancer risk by half.[3] When combined with PBM, it lowers overall breast cancer risk by 95 percent and offers an additional benefit: if you do develop breast cancer after BSO, your odds of a second diagnosis are cut in half as well (table 5.1).[4] Like PBM, the decision to have BSO should be made only after careful consideration, because it can cause serious side effects: if you're still having menstrual periods, it will push your body into menopause and you may have to prematurely contend with hot flashes, insomnia, vaginal dryness, and other change-of-life symptoms. Your gynecologist or oncologist can discuss these issues with you and let you know what to expect.

Even with its impressive risk-reducing benefit, PBM is a deeply personal choice. It isn't right for everyone, and it shouldn't be considered lightly, because once done, it can't be undone. On the other hand, if you're prepared to do whatever you can to reduce your high chance of being diagnosed with breast cancer and dealing with surgery, chemotherapy, or radiation, it's your most effective alternative. PBM may be an easy decision for some women. Others would never consider removing their healthy breasts. Whatever your circumstances, the decision can be torturous. Should you? Shouldn't you? No one can answer that question for you.

If you decide PBM is the best way to have peace of mind as you live your life, you'll be a candidate for skin-sparing or nipple-sparing mastectomies with immediate reconstruction. From a cosmetic standpoint, reconstruction after PBM produces some of the very best results, particularly if your healthy breasts are unscarred from biopsies or previous surgeries. If you're unsatisfied with the shape, size, or position of your natural breasts, those issues may be corrected with reconstruction, even though your new breasts won't have the same sensation.

> *My mother has breast cancer again; one of her sisters is in stage 4, another is in remission. My grandmother and the rest of my mother's sisters died of cancer. Even with this history, having my breasts removed was the hardest decision I've ever had to make. Though I had many breakdowns, I knew after all the crying that the decision I made was the right one. My breasts were precious to me but not as precious as my children. I wanted to make sure I'll be here to see them go off to life. Believe me when I say it's a relief.*   —Nora

> *I do think PBM is pretty extreme, but so is cancer. It's all a matter of how much risk you are willing to live with day to day, compared to your willingness to undergo major surgery to reduce that risk to as close to zero as possible. You do as much research as you can by reading and talking to people who have the appropriate knowledge and experience, then you do what's right for you. I didn't want PBM. However, in examining my own personal and family history, my temperament, and life goals, I couldn't not have it.*   —Jill

Contralateral mastectomy. Women who face unilateral mastectomy sometimes choose to also remove their healthy breast with a *contralateral mastectomy*, to eliminate most of the potential for being diagnosed with cancer again in the future. Contralateral mastectomy isn't recommended for most breast cancer patients, because the chance of a future diagnosis is low, less than 1 percent per year. Your odds are increased if your breast cancer occurs in more than one spot in your breast, if you have invasive lobular cancer, or if you have a BRCA gene mutation. Rates of contralateral mastectomies have increased in recent years, perhaps in part because more women now have pre-mastectomy MRIs, which sometimes show early-stage abnormalities in the opposite breast. Even though an MRI may produce false positive results, women who have pre-mastectomy MRIs choose contralateral mastectomy twice as often as those who don't.[5]

Reconstruction may also be a deciding factor; better symmetry is more likely when both breasts are removed and reconstructed at the same time. For some, particularly those who would like to retain at least one breast with normal sensation, removing their remaining, healthy breast may be unacceptable. If you're facing unilateral mastectomy, having an accurate perception of your risk will help you decide whether you should remove the contralateral breast as well.

Unless you've walked in my BRCA shoes . . . Ultimately, whether you proceed with prophylactic mastectomy is your decision, but everyone you know will have an opinion about what you should or shouldn't do. Friends and family might consider breast removal to be extreme. Unless they've had to make the decision themselves, people may not comprehend why you would deliberately remove your perfectly healthy breasts. They might not understand that while you would certainly prefer to keep your breasts, you view them as life-threatening enemies.

Take the time you need to consider what each risk-reducing option involves, how it affects your current and future level of risk, and the potential side effects. Speak with your health care team, including a genetics specialist, to gain a clear sense of your own risk. Carefully consider your tolerance for risk, your lifestyle, and other factors before deciding which alternative is the best decision for you. Visit FORCE (www.facingourrisk .org), the most comprehensive source of information for anyone who is genetically predisposed to breast or ovarian cancer. Helpline support is available by phone, and the organization's message boards offer a supportive, safe, and empowering place to learn, share, and just vent about genetic high risk, prophylactic surgery, and reconstruction. *Confronting Hereditary Breast and Ovarian Cancer*, the organization's decision-making resource for previvors and *survivors* of hereditary cancer, is a comprehensive roadmap for living in a high-risk body.

Paying for Preventive High-Risk Services

The Patient Protection and Affordable Care Act of 2010 (more simply known as the Affordable Care Act) requires health care plans or policies issued on or after March 23, 2010, to cover chemoprevention counseling and certain other preventive services at no cost to patients. (The law does not apply to genetic testing.) Included within these guidelines is genetic counseling for individuals whose family history indicates a potential increased risk for a BRCA mutation. Your policy may require you to use in-network professionals; it cannot require deductibles or co-payments for these services. Some plans are exempt. Visit Healthcare.gov (www.health care.gov) for more details and information about other preventive services that are included in the no-cost category. You'll read about insurance coverage of PBM in chapter 18.

PART TWO ○ RECONSTRUCTIVE PROCEDURES

CHAPTER SIX

Breast Implants

One doesn't discover new lands without consenting to lose sight of the shore for a very long time.

—ANDRÉ GIDE, WINNER OF THE
1947 NOBEL PRIZE IN LITERATURE

Before tissue flap surgery, implants were the only method of reconstructing breasts after mastectomy. Implant reconstruction is the simplest method of recreating breasts, and compared with tissue flap procedures, the surgery is shorter and leaves fewer scars. Recovery is faster, but the traditional overall reconstruction process takes longer to complete.

Implant reconstruction is a good option if you:

- don't have an active infection anywhere in your body
- aren't pregnant or nursing
- don't want to scar additional parts of your body
- don't have enough fat for a tissue flap reconstruction
- can't endure a lengthier flap reconstruction operation
- are willing to surgically alter your healthy breast to achieve symmetry (if you're having unilateral mastectomy with reconstruction)

Defining Your New Breasts

Implant reconstruction involves several decisions that are best made during consultation with your plastic surgeon, who will describe where your incisions will be made and explain the different types of implants available to you.

Implants inside and out. Breast implants are filled with either *saline* (sterile salt water) or *silicone* gel. A breast reconstructed with a saline implant doesn't have the softness, resilience, and bounce of silicone gel, which behaves and feels more like natural breast tissue. In the 1970s and 1980s, silicone implants were filled with a thin silicone gel. Newer-generation models contain *cohesive gel* with a consistency like Jell-O; this provides a firm yet soft implant that maintains its shape and is less likely to leak if the shell ruptures. All implants, including those filled with saline, have outer shells of silicone elastomer, a thin medical-grade rubber, similar to the material used in heart shunts, pacemakers, and artificial limbs.

During your consultation appointment, ask your plastic surgeon for samples of saline and silicone implants so you can compare how they feel (some surgeons prefer to use only saline, and others use only silicone), and request a copy of the implant product information; the same information is also available on the implant manufacturer's website. Consider speaking with other patients who have had implant reconstruction (your plastic surgeon can put you in touch), so you'll have the benefit of their experience. Some may even be willing to give you a peek or a poke at their results. If you're contemplating breast implants, consider the differences between silicone and saline before you make your final decision about how your reconstruction will be done (table 6.1).

Saline implants are either round or contoured (figure 6.1). Silicone implants are always round—eventually, contoured silicone implants will

TABLE 6.1. Comparing saline and silicone implants

Characteristic	Saline implant	Silicone implant
Components	Silicone shell filled with salt water	Silicone shell with silicone gel interior
Texture	Not as soft as silicone	Soft, like natural breast tissue
Incision required	Shorter (implant is deflated when inserted)	Longer (implant is full when inserted)
Interior substance	Filled by surgeon during operation	Pre-filled by manufacturer
Rupture	Obvious	May be undetected
Follow-up recommended	None	Periodic MRI screening

probably be available as well. Round implants are used most often for reconstruction in the United States. They create fullness across the breast. When you stand or sit, the saline collects in the lower portion of the implant, providing a natural slope to the breast. When you lie flat, it moves to the outside of the breast, just as natural tissue does. Contoured implants are longer and narrower, with more fullness at the bottom. You might think they would provide a more natural shape, but they aren't the best solution for every woman. Your chest structure and the elasticity of your breast skin influence the shape of your new breast as much as, if

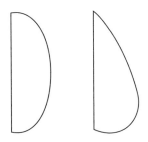

FIGURE 6.1. Implants are either round (*left*) or contoured (*right*). Saline implants are available in both shapes; all silicone implants are round.

not more than, the type of implant used. Contoured implants have a rough or textured exterior to keep them from shifting or flipping over once they're in place; some round implants are also textured. Texturing was developed to discourage *capsular contracture*, hard scar tissue that forms around the implant and can distort its shape. This doesn't always work, however, and rippling—the appearance of indentations that look like small waves under the skin—occurs more frequently in the outer shell of textured implants. Your plastic surgeon will help you decide which shape and type of implant is best for you.

Size and projection. Communicating how big or small you'd like your new breasts to be isn't as easy as saying "make me a 36B," because implant volume doesn't readily translate to bra size. Implant capacity is measured in cubic centimeters (cc): 30 cc of saline equals one ounce. Your physical characteristics make all the difference in how a particular implant looks in proportion to the rest of your body: a 480 cc implant will look much larger on a 5' 4" woman who weighs 120 pounds than on a woman who is 5' 9" and weighs 160 pounds.

If you are having *unilateral reconstruction*, your surgeon will choose an implant that closely matches the size of your opposite breast. With *bilateral reconstruction*, you have a clean slate for new breasts that are smaller or bigger than your natural breasts or of similar size. Choosing the right size is important: implants that are too small won't give you the cleavage you want; if they're too large, they might upset your body's aesthetic proportions.

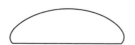 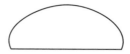 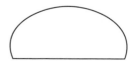

FIGURE 6.2. Implants are available in different widths, volumes, and profiles.

Many women leave the choice of implants to their surgeons. However, the size of your reconstructed breast shouldn't be a surprise when you wake up from surgery. It should be a topic that you and your surgeon discuss before you enter the operating room. By actively participating in the decision, you're more likely to be satisfied with the size of your reconstructed breasts—dissatisfaction with size is a common reason for replacing implants—so it's a good idea to be sure you and your surgeon are on the same page about what you want. Once you decide whether you prefer saline or silicone, your surgeon will select implants that fit the diameter of your chest wall and, among those, will choose an implant that provides the volume and projection you want. If you're large-framed, low- or moderate-profile implants, which are wider at the base, will provide a better fit than high-profile implants that have more projection but are designed to fit women with a narrow chest (figure 6.2). Saline implants tend to offer more projection, because they're more rigid than silicone implants.

ADVANTAGES OF IMPLANT RECONSTRUCTION
- *Surgery to place an implant is shorter and less complex than tissue flap reconstruction.*
- *It uses the mastectomy incision for reconstruction (it doesn't create additional scarring).*
- *The procedure can be completed in one step when combined with nipple-sparing mastectomy (if no revisions are required).*
- *It is a viable alternative for women who don't want or can't have flap reconstruction.*
- *Future weight changes won't affect the size of your new breasts.*
- *It's easy to find qualified surgeons.*

DISADVANTAGES OF IMPLANT RECONSTRUCTION
- *The overall reconstruction process can be much longer than a tissue flap procedure.*

- *Most procedures involve multiple steps and multiple office visits.*
- *The new breast doesn't always feel, look, or move like a natural breast.*
- *The implant is subject to rupture, deflation, capsular contracture, and other inherent problems.*
- *Surgical modification of the healthy breast (if you have unilateral reconstruction) is usually needed to achieve symmetry.*
- *Results are often poor when breast skin has undergone radiation.*
- *Implants don't last a lifetime.*

Are They Safe?

Breast implants have been around in one form or another for decades. First-generation silicone implants were developed in 1961 by two plastic surgeons and the Dow Corning Corporation; saline implants were introduced two years later. Within a few years, breast augmentation was a booming business, and several manufacturers were mass-producing implants to meet rapidly growing demand. By the time the U.S. Food and Drug Administration (FDA) began regulating implants in 1976, thousands of women already had them.

More than 9,000 individual and class action suits were filed in the early 1990s against Dow and other implant manufacturers, claiming silicone implants caused arthritis, immune system disorders, and a host of other health problems. Implant companies and plastic surgeons were caught between a rock and a hard place: though implants had been used for 30 years, their long-term safety had never been established. Dow ultimately lost the court cases and filed for bankruptcy. In 1992, the FDA banned the use of silicone implants for cosmetic purposes, reclassified them as experimental, and approved their use only for breast reconstruction and clinical studies, until manufacturers could prove the devices were safe. Five years later, the FDA-chartered Institute of Medicine (IOM) reviewed all past and ongoing scientific research related to the safety of silicone breast implants. No evidence linking implants to cancer, other disease, or any other significant health problems was found. Subsequent studies in the United States, Canada, and Europe concurred.

The IOM did identify the following local problems (confined to the breast) with both saline and silicone implants:

- Complications are not uncommon. According to the FDA, most women with implants can expect to have at least one complication in the three years following their initial implant surgery; half of them require at least one subsequent operation within seven years.[1]
- Medical intervention, including surgery, is often needed to address problems.
- Implants don't last forever. Sooner or later, they need to be replaced.

The ban remained in effect until the FDA recognized numerous large-scale studies that showed no cause-and-effect relationship between silicone implants and serious health issues. In 2006, the FDA conditionally approved silicone implants, directing the two U.S. manufacturers, Mentor and McGhan, to study 80,000 women with the devices over 10 years (McGhan subsequently became Inamed and is now Allergan, the company that also markets Botox). The FDA approved silicone implants from a third company, Sientra, in 2012. All silicone implants now used in the United States are also subject to the FDA's Medical Device Tracking regulations; surgeons must forward certain patient data to the FDA, so that every woman who has a silicone implant becomes part of a national database that is used to track and evaluate problems.

Do implants cause disease? Silicone implants are the most studied medical devices in the history of medicine, and two decades after the landmark litigation against Dow Corning, they're considered to be safe. A small percentage of women with silicone implants develop characteristics of lupus, psoriasis, chronic fatigue syndrome, rheumatoid arthritis, and other autoimmune conditions. Some scientists explain the connection this way: more than two million women in this country have implants. Inevitably, autoimmune problems will occur in a population of that size, with or without implants. In other words, autoimmune disease symptoms occur no more frequently in women with silicone implants than in those without the devices. Even though most physicians consider silicone implants to be safe and there is no significant evidence to the contrary, some experts still contend that silicone may be problematic for women who already have weakened immune systems. FDA-required patient information states that the "safety and effectiveness have not been established in patients with auto immune diseases (for example, lupus and scleroderma) or a weakened immune system."

The FDA issued an advisory in 2011 about "a possible association between breast implants and the development of anaplastic large cell lymphoma (ALCL), a rare type of non-Hodgkin's lymphoma," and stated that "women with breast implants may have a very low albeit increased risk of developing ALCL adjacent to the breast implant."[2] ALCL isn't a breast cancer; it's a systemic disease that may occur in the surrounding scar tissue. The agency identified the risk as very small: about 60 cases among the 5 to 10 million women worldwide who have saline or silicone implants. Until more data are available, the FDA recommends seeing a physician if the area around an implant looks or feels unusual.

Tissue Expander-to-Implant Reconstruction

When implants are used to augment the size of healthy breasts, they can be placed over or under the pectoralis muscle. With reconstruction, implants are most often placed behind the *pectoralis major* muscle, the muscle bodybuilders like to bulk up. Because there is little remaining breast tissue after mastectomy, the muscle provides a cushioning layer between the skin and the implant. Before implants can be placed into the chest, however, a pocket must be created to hold them in place. For most women who choose implant reconstruction, the process involves two separate stages several months apart. (Figure 6.3 shows the timelines for the several types of implant reconstruction.)

Creating a pocket. Working through the mastectomy incision, the surgeon detaches the lower edge of the muscle from the chest wall, then lifts up the muscle and shapes a pocket behind it. Because most women don't have quite enough skin after mastectomy to adequately hold a full-sized implant, a temporary implant called a *tissue expander* is placed in the pocket and partially filled with 60 to 100 cc of saline (some surgeons prefer to add more saline at this stage). This pushes the muscle forward, creating a little bulge. The muscle edge is pulled down over the upper portion of the expander. The incision is then closed with dissolvable stitches and surgical tape. The process takes about an hour for each breast. When you wake up, you'll have starter breast mounds, so your chest won't be completely flat.

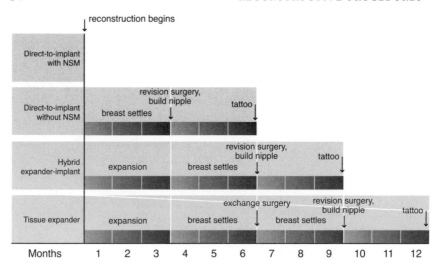

FIGURE 6.3. Implant reconstruction timeline. Intervals may differ, depending on breast cancer treatment, the preference of patient and surgeon, and complications that may delay completion.

Expansion and implant exchange. Within two or three weeks, when your chest has healed sufficiently, you'll begin getting saline "fills" in your surgeon's office. The expander will slowly inflate like a balloon each time more saline is added. The chest muscle thins until it pushes against the front of the breast, and the space behind the muscle grows. The breast skin also stretches, similar to the way a woman's abdominal skin expands during pregnancy. (The expansion process is described in more detail in chapter 7.) When the pocket is large enough, your expander is replaced with a softer and better-shaped saline or silicone implant (also described in chapter 7).

Once your implant has had time to settle into place (at least three months after stage 2, the exchange surgery), your new nipple can be created in a short operation (described in chapter 11). Cosmetic revisions, if required, can also be performed at this stage. The final, separate step in the reconstructive process adds color to the nipple and simulates the areola (see chapter 11).

Direct-to-Implant Reconstruction

Direct-to-implant reconstruction (also called *non-expansive, one-step,* and *single-stage* implant reconstruction) places a full-sized implant into the pocket immediately after mastectomy, eliminating altogether the need for expansion. Unless complications occur or revisions are necessary, this skip-a-step procedure completes the entire "invisible" reconstruction during a single visit to the operating room. The process is made possible with nipple-sparing mastectomy (you keep your own nipples, so there is no need to recreate them) com-

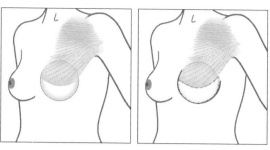

FIGURE 6.4. In traditional implant reconstruction, the pectoralis muscle typically covers only the upper part of the implant (*left*). Adding a patch of acellular dermal matrix along the lower edge of the muscle (*right*) provides complete coverage.

bined with an *acellular dermal matrix (ADM),* a tissue substitute made from human skin that has been stripped of its cells but still has collagen and other proteins. Originally developed as a source of *skin grafts* for burn victims, acellular material is organic; it provides a biological framework that supports the growth of new blood vessels. AlloDerm may be the best known ADM product; other, similar products, including Tutoplast, DermaMatrix, Strattice (from pig skin), and others, are also used and are regulated by the FDA.

Acellular dermal matrix benefits implant reconstruction in several ways. In traditional implant reconstruction, the pectoralis muscle isn't broad enough to completely cover the lower portion of the implant (figure 6.4). Tacking a patch of ADM along the edge of the pectoralis muscle covers the lower portion of the implant, forming an instant pocket and defining the inframammary crease, completing in a single procedure what expansion achieves over several months. The ADM smooths contour, cushions the skin from direct contact with the implant, and provides an internal sling that holds the implant in position.

If direct-to-implant reconstruction (figure 6.5) sounds right for you, consider the following:

- Most surgeons still prefer the tried-and-true expansion process, so it may be difficult to find someone who offers this type of reconstruction.
- Choose a plastic surgeon who is well experienced with the procedure.
- Many plastic surgeons now use ADM with traditional expansion reconstruction, so be sure to clarify whether a particular surgeon performs direct-to-implant reconstruction.

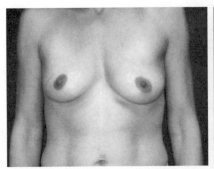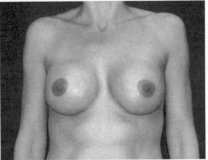

FIGURE 6.5. Before (*left*) and after (*right*) bilateral nipple-sparing mastectomy with immediate direct-to-implant reconstruction. *Images provided by C. Andrew Salzberg, M.D.*

- A reconstruction that begins as direct-to-implant reconstruction may require additional procedures, if revision surgery is needed to correct problems or improve cosmetic results.
- Ask your plastic surgeon whether you're a candidate for direct-to-implant reconstruction.

Choosing preventive mastectomy to reduce my inherited risk for breast cancer was a difficult decision. I did not think I would be able to look in the mirror if I had no reconstruction, but I knew I did not want to have fat removed from other parts of my body and endure more scars and healing time. I wanted my reconstruction to be over and done; I did not want to have to go back for fills and more surgery. Then I discovered nipple-sparing mastectomy with direct-to-implant reconstruction. The surgery was minimal and recovery was short. My procedure was a success and three or four weeks later, I felt very good. I was an A-cup before my mastectomy; now I am a B-cup. I look so much better than before, and I have sensation toward the outer parts of my breasts. My nipples react to cold, yet I have no feeling on or around them. I love the results.   —Leslie

Other direct-to-implant procedures. Two other immediate reconstructive procedures are exceptions to the traditional expansion process. Some small-breasted women may have enough skin after mastectomy to accommodate a fixed-volume implant right away, without expansion or exchange procedures. Women who have immediate reconstruction with an implant that is covered with tissue from their back (described in chapter 9) also skip the need for exchange surgery.

What happens if you have augmented breasts at the time of mastectomy? Most surgeons would probably remove the implant before proceeding with the mastectomy, and then continue with implant reconstruction, if that is your choice. Some surgeons are experimenting with a different procedure that leaves the implant in place while your breast tissue is removed. Once the mastectomy is complete, the old implant is replaced with a new one. This "implant-sparing mastectomy" is by no means standard procedure; it was developed in recognition of the many women who have breast augmentation before their breast cancer diagnosis (breast augmentation is the most commonly performed cosmetic surgery).[3]

Recovery

After implant reconstruction, your breast area will be numb and may feel heavy or ache for a few days. If lymph nodes were removed during your surgery, your underarm may also be numb or sore. Any discomfort will be controlled by pain medication. You'll be encouraged to get up and begin walking the day after your surgery; you should take progressively longer walks each day. After your operation, you'll be able to carefully lift your arms to wash your face and brush your teeth. It will take another week or more before you can lift them over your head. You'll be very tired and sore for a couple of weeks, but your strength will slowly return. Each day, you'll spend more time awake and less time napping. You'll be back to most of your normal routine in two to three weeks; you may need to restrict upper body motion for a week or two longer, and for several months you should avoid strenuous activities and movements that pull excessively on the muscle. (Table 6.2 summarizes the timetable for the reconstructive procedures and recovery.)

Before reconstruction, you may wonder whether you'll always be conscious of your implants. Will they ever feel a part of you, as your natural breasts did? They may feel heavy at first, and you'll feel them shift in the pocket when you stretch or lift and move when your chest muscles flex or contract. This shouldn't be painful, although it can feel odd until you

TABLE 6.2. Intervals for implant reconstruction and recovery

Procedure	Surgery and hospital stay	Most routine activities resumed
Expanders	About 1 hour per breast; usually 1 day in hospital*	At 2–3 weeks
Exchange surgery	Up to 1 hour per breast; outpatient	At 1 week
Direct-to-implant	About 1 hour per breast; 1–2 days in hospital*	At 2–3 weeks

Note: Reflects bilateral reconstruction without complications. Surgical expertise and individual healing affect recovery times.
*Delayed reconstruction can be performed as an outpatient procedure.

become accustomed to it. After several months, your implants will become softer, feel more natural, and drop into a more natural position on your chest. You'll get used to them in time.

Bras are optional after implant reconstruction. Even though you won't need one, you might enjoy wearing pretty lingerie after reconstruction. If you decide to shop for new bras, you might need a different size than you wore before your mastectomy, because your new breast or breasts may not have the same shape, size, or projection. You may be limited to wearing seamless stretch bras if your breast doesn't project enough to fill a regular bra cup. After unilateral reconstruction, it may be difficult to find a bra that fits both breasts correctly.

Potential Problems

Though most women who have implants are quite satisfied, complications, including many that require revision surgery, are not uncommon. Implant manufacturers provide information about complications, how often they occur, and reasons for reoperation; you can find this online (www.your breastoptions.com and www.Natrelle.com) and in the printed disclaimer included in the implant packaging (ask for this during your consultation with your plastic surgeon).

Ruptures and leaks. A *rupture* is a tear in the outer shell of an implant that can result from injury to the breast, normal aging of the implant, or other reasons. Improved manufacturing standards and quality have decreased the frequency of ruptures and leaks, yet they can still occur. If a saline implant leaks, you'll know it, because your reconstructed breast will deflate in a very obvious way in a day or two (figure 6.6). The body safely absorbs the harmless saline, but the implant

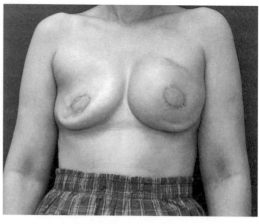

FIGURE 6.6. Although a silicone rupture may go unnoticed, a saline implant rupture, as shown here, is obvious. *Image provided by Gail S. Lebovic, MA, MD, FACS.*

must be removed. When a silicone implant ruptures, you might feel a hard knot; have breast pain, swelling, or numbness; or notice a change in your breast size or shape. Because the cohesive gel usually remains in the pocket or scar capsule around it, however, you may be unaware of the rupture. If an MRI, ultrasound, or *computed tomography (CT)* scan shows that the implant has indeed ruptured, it must be removed and can then be replaced. Because there are often no visual changes to indicate the *silent rupture* of a silicone implant, the FDA recommends an MRI three years after your initial implant surgery and every two years thereafter (your health insurance may not pay for these screenings). If you'd like to see how punctures or ruptures affect saline and silicone implants, visit YouTube (www.youtube .com) and search for "breast implant rupture."

Newer-generation "gummy bear" silicone implants have stronger shells and a thicker cohesive gel filler. Unlike older silicone implants, a gummy bear implant has an interior that is surrounded by three shell layers, so it's firmer than other silicone implants (but still soft) and is expected to last longer with fewer complications. These have been available in Europe and Latin America for several years, and their safety and durability is well documented. Currently, gummy bear implants are in *clinical trials* in the United States; it's probably just a matter of time before they're approved by the FDA.

The Ideal implant (www.idealimplant.com) features a unique design of saline-filled chambers that are nested together. Developed with input

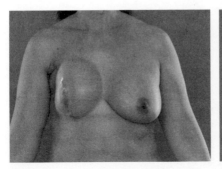 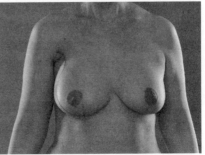

FIGURE 6.7. Capsular contracture may distort breast shape (*left*). This delayed reconstruction was salvaged by removing the scar tissue and replacing the implant with a tissue flap (*right*). *Images provided by Dr. Frank J. DellaCroce and The Center for Restorative Breast Surgery, LLC.*

from plastic surgeons, the Ideal is meant to decrease ruptures and wrinkles, while providing a more natural feel, much like a silicone implant. If these investigational implants prove successful during clinical trials and obtain FDA approval, they may eventually become another reconstructive alternative for women.

Capsular contracture. After reconstruction, a capsule of scar tissue forms around the implant. This isn't unusual and it isn't a health hazard. It is the body's natural reaction to foreign matter and also occurs in patients who have pacemakers, artificial hips, or other types of implants. Capsular contracture—the most common reason for reoperation after implant reconstruction—occurs when the scar tissue tightens and squeezes the implant. Mild capsular contracture (grades I and II) may cause the breast to feel more firm without affecting its appearance. More severe cases (grades III and IV) can be painful and distort the breast (figure 6.7). The condition develops more commonly in smokers and in women who have had radiation therapy, though it's a mystery why some women experience capsular contracture repeatedly and others never have it. It can develop within a few months of reconstruction or years later.

When capsular contracture develops, the remedy usually involves surgery. In some cases, a *capsulectomy* can be performed to cut scar tissue away from the implant. (*Capsulotomy*, trying to break the capsule by squeezing it, isn't recommended.) For most women, however, the implant must be removed and replaced—using ADM with a replacement implant may help reduce the chances of another capsular contracture, but there's no guarantee it won't happen again. Limited evidence shows that using ADM with immediate direct-to-implant reconstruction lowers the rate of capsular contracture within eight years of reconstruction to less than 0.5 percent.[4]

Regularly massaging your implants may help discourage the formation of additional scar tissue; your surgeon will show you the proper method to do this. It's somewhat easier when you have round, smooth saline implants, which can be moved around in the pocket more than textured or contoured implants. If you develop capsular contracture, your surgeon may prescribe lymphatic breast massage, ultrasound, or vitamin E to soften the scar tissue. Muscle relaxants may also help. More surgeons are taking a preventive approach to reducing infection around the implant, which is known to cause capsular contracture, by using a "no touch technique." Before placing the implant into the pocket, the surgeon changes his surgical gown and bathes his gloves, surgical instruments, and the implant in antibiotic liquid. The pocket is also flushed with antibiotic fluid. The aim is to reduce the level of bacteria that may be on the surface of the implant when it goes under the muscle. Anecdotal evidence from plastic surgeons shows that the procedure does reduce the incidence of capsular contracture.

Rippling or wrinkling. You may be able to feel or see ripples and wrinkles in the implant, especially if your breast skin is thin. Corrective measures include placing the implant under the muscle (if it was previously over the muscle), replacing a textured implant with one that is smooth, or adding a layer of ADM between the implant and the skin. Saline implants more frequently show ripples and wrinkles, and for that reason they are routinely overfilled to decrease the likelihood of this occurring—but this also makes the implant more firm. Each implant has a range for overfilling set by the manufacturer; exceeding these limits can affect its durability and may void the warranty. That is one reason why, if your implant is smaller than you would like, it's a better idea for your plastic surgeon to swap it for a somewhat larger one than overfill beyond the manufacturer's advised range.

Gel bleed. In some cases, when a silicone implant ruptures, oil in the cohesive gel can leech through the implant shell into the surrounding capsule of scar tissue and may invade the lymph nodes. Although not as common, gel oil can also migrate to distant organs. It's not obvious when this happens, unless lymph nodes become enlarged or appear unusual during a subsequent surgery. The implant and scar tissue around it must then be removed. Although the newer cohesive gel implants have tougher shells and appear to be more durable, MRI studies of Danish women found that the gel migrated beyond the scar capsule in three-quarters of women who had implant ruptures.[5] FDA investigations have shown no evidence of harm from silicone exposure, and a 1999 IOM report determined that human exposure to silicones, even at high doses, doesn't cause serious or long-term health problems. Silicone is a synthetic substance manufactured by combining certain chemical substances with silicon, the second most common natural chemical element on the planet. Silicon is ubiquitous in the environment; we're all exposed to it as a part of modern life. It's used in thousands of everyday products, including cosmetics, nonstick cookware, and even antacids. It's commonly found in small amounts in the body, including in breast milk, even in individuals who don't have silicone implants.

Cosmetic issues. While any reconstructive surgery has the potential for cosmetic problems, some are unique to implants. All cosmetic issues can be improved and many can be eliminated, although additional surgery may be required.

Asymmetry is common and is typically corrected by replacing the implants. After unilateral reconstruction, it can be difficult to match your natural breast without additional surgery, because implants can't be shaped and sculpted like living tissue. You may become asymmetrical over time, because your implanted breast won't droop or reflect weight changes, as your natural breast does.

Malpositioned implants move too far up, down, or to the sides of the pocket. If the skin stretches too much, an implant can "bottom out," moving below the inframammary crease. Patches of ADM can be added beneath or along the sides of the implant to improve its positioning and keep it where it belongs.

Implant movement can be excessive if the pocket is too large. One method of repair is to return to the operating room to remove the implant and surgically reduce the size of the pocket. If the movement isn't excessive, an easier fix is to place a small ADM graft around the implant, reducing the space between the implant and the pocket.

The weight of the implant may stretch the skin until the implant *extrudes* or comes through the skin, particularly in women who smoke or have thin or irradiated skin. When this occurs, the implant has to be removed and the skin allowed to heal before a new implant can be placed.

Symmastia occurs when the pockets on either side are too close together, eliminating the natural space between the breasts—the breasts look as though they're joined in the middle, creating a condition that women sometimes refer to as "uniboob." This results from cutting too much of the muscle when the pockets are formed or using implants that are too big or too wide. Repair involves reducing the pocket size or reinforcing the inside borders of the pockets with ADM to hold the implants in proper position.

Insufficient cleavage may be improved with fat injections or by using somewhat larger or wider implants.

Removing or replacing your implant. Like washing machines, tires, and other manufactured products, implants eventually wear out. There's no way to predict how long yours will last, although improvements continue to be made and newer implants are expected to last longer. Some women have implants for 10 to 20 years without complication, but most women will need to have them replaced at least once during their lifetime. This risk of replacement increases as the implant ages. To put this in perspective: pacemakers must be replaced every few years. Perhaps that's the best way to view implants.

Unless complications occur, it's not particularly difficult to replace an implant. The pocket is already there, so most of the work is done. The surgeon accesses the pocket through the mastectomy incision, removes any excess scar tissue, and swaps the old implant with a new one. Generally, implants can be replaced in an *outpatient procedure* taking just an hour or so for each implant, with minimal discomfort. If you decide not to replace your implants, you can opt for reconstruction with your own tissue. If you prefer to forgo any additional reconstruction, most of your breast skin will be removed and you'll have a slanting scar across your chest, as though you had a mastectomy without reconstruction.

No matter how simple it may be to replace an implant, the process can be emotionally disruptive: you're happily living your post-mastectomy life, then you must undergo more doctor visits and additional surgery to repair a problem with your new breast. Some women say it's like reliving their reconstruction all over again. Other women consider replacement surgery a price they're willing to pay. Either way, it's an important consideration when deciding which technique is best for you.

> *I don't mind if the implant must be exchanged in the future. I consider it required maintenance, like getting my car serviced. I can take time every few years to do that if I need to. Besides, maybe they'll have something better by then and I can trade up to a better model!*   *—Belle*

Implant warranties. Before your initial surgery, your doctor or one of the office staff should give you a copy of the manufacturer's implant warranty and explain its terms. (You can also read the warranty terms online at the manufacturer's website.) Once your implants are in place, be sure you have your implant ID card before you leave the hospital. Your nurse should provide a copy of the warranty for you, which lists the brand, type, size, and serial numbers of your implants. You'll need this information to activate your warranty. Mentor and Allergan offer 10-year guarantees: if your implant develops a rupture or other qualifying event within that time, the company will replace it at no charge and provide limited financial assistance to defray related hospital and surgical costs not covered by health insurance. Extended warranties are also available.

CHAPTER SEVEN

The Expander Experience

The way I see it, if you want the rainbow, you gotta be willing to put up with the rain. —DOLLY PARTON

Tissue expanders deserve an entire chapter to themselves because, if you decide to reconstruct your breasts with implants, it's the process most plastic surgeons prefer. Although it can be tedious, expansion is an amazing process. A helpful illustrated, step-by-step photo journal of expansion is available at "Myself: Together Again" (www.myselftogetheragain.org).

Getting Your Fill

Two or three weeks after your initial surgery, you'll begin regular visits to your plastic surgeon's office to gradually fill your expanders. She'll use a magnetic device, like a mini version of a carpenter's stud finder, to locate the internal port on the front of the expander, just under your skin—you may be able to feel it if you run your fingers over your breast skin. (Some expanders have a remote valve outside the skin.) Each fill appointment takes only a few minutes. Your surgeon will inject 50 to 120 cc (about 3.5 to 8 tablespoons) of sterile saline into the expander through the port (figure 7.1).

You probably won't feel the needle, because it's quite small and your breast will be numb, although some women say the needle feels like a bee sting. Every week or two, you'll return to repeat the process.

You'll begin to see significant changes with each

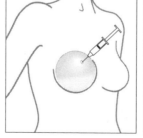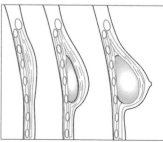

FIGURE 7.1. Adding saline to the tissue expander (*left*) gradually stretches the muscle and surrounding skin, until the flat mastectomy site slowly grows into a fully formed breast mound (*right*).

TABLE 7.1. Sample intervals for tissue expansion

Total volume of implant (cc)

Volume added at biweekly fill (cc)*	6 weeks	8 weeks	10 weeks	12 weeks
60	240	300	360	420
100	360	460	560	660
140	480	620	—	—

*Assumptions: 60 cc added at initial surgery; each fill adds equal amount of saline.

fill, as your cleavage develops and the inframammary fold forms under your breast. During your last one or two appointments, your expander will be somewhat overfilled. This ensures that you'll have sufficient skin to cover your implant and enough space so the implant will sit low in the pocket with a more natural droop, instead of unnaturally high on your chest. For most women, the expanders are completely filled in six to eight weeks. Your own interval may be shorter or longer, depending on how much your skin must stretch to accommodate an implant and how well you tolerate the process (table 7.1). If your plastic surgeon uses an acellular dermal matrix with the tissue expander, she can introduce more saline during the initial operation. You'll then require fewer subsequent fills, and your expansion can be completed sooner. If you're having chemotherapy treatments during expansion, talk to your doctor about the best time to get your fills. It may be helpful to schedule your expansion fills a day or two before your chemotherapy, when your resistance to infection is strongest.

Minimizing Your Discomfort

Expanders are built for function, not for comfort. Some women sail through the process with minimal discomfort, while others find it irritating, stressful, and very uncomfortable. At the very least, the lower portion of your chest where the muscles are attached to the ribs will feel tight. Your chest may feel heavy or tender, particularly if you had radiation therapy before your reconstruction. It may ache, as though you've done many more pushups than you should have. Your chest will feel tighter and fuller each time more saline is added, but the feeling will subside somewhat after a couple of days. It's a bit like having dental braces: just when you get used to them, the dentist tightens them, and they're uncomfortable all over again. Your muscles may also contract and sometimes spasm as they stretch between fills. One day, though, the muscles will relax and you'll feel much better. Try the following tips to relieve your discomfort:

- Pain medication isn't usually required during fills. However, if the process is too uncomfortable, try taking acetaminophen (Tylenol) immediately before or after your fills. If that doesn't do the trick, ask your surgeon to prescribe a muscle relaxant, anti-inflammatory, or pain medication.
- Take warm (not hot) showers, or soak a towel or washcloth in very warm water, wring it out, and hold it against your ribcage. Don't use a heating pad on your mastectomy site—with your post-mastectomy numbness, you won't feel the heat and you may be unaware if your skin begins to burn.
- Gentle massage relaxes the muscles and provides temporary relief. Apply oil or lotion and rub along the side and front of the rib cage several times a day. Or ask your surgeon for a referral to a physical therapist, who can massage and relax the connective tissues in your chest.
- Exercise is beneficial during expansion, as long as it doesn't involve high-impact activities such as aerobics, jogging, or swimming until your surgeon says it's okay to do so. Avoid lifting weights or other activities that increase or strengthen your pectoralis muscles, so it won't become more difficult to stretch them.
- If your expansion is unbearable, ask your surgeon to remove some saline from your expander, allow more time between fills, or add less saline each time. You'll be eager to be done with the process, but take time to listen to your body; it will be worth it in the long run. Or consider having Botox injected directly into the chest muscle: small trials show that women who had injections suffered fewer muscle spasms, needed less pain medication during expansion, and tolerated larger fills.[1]

I had an amazing experience with tissue expanders without any real complications. The pain was brutal at times, but was mostly relieved with medication. Staying on top of pain meds, resting when needed, and using muscle relaxants made it very doable. I was excited to watch the "growing" process unfold each week. I was truly in awe after each fill, despite the tightness that occurred a few hours later and continued through the evening. However, the next day I felt well again. I resumed gym activities after my first expansion and my exchange surgery went off without a hitch. I returned to full-time work five weeks after my mastectomy. Tissue expanders are not for everyone, but they can be a positive experience for those who go into the procedure knowing what to expect from the process.   —Lenore

Once I scheduled my mastectomy and tissue expander surgery, I had plenty of time to worry. I spent hours on the Internet reading about it. I also watched videos about women going through expansion and they made the fills seem so painful! The first time I had a fill I was pretty nervous. Honestly, I felt the first contact the needle had with my skin, almost like a bug bite. After that, the only discomfort was at the end, when the muscle and skin stretched. I took Tylenol before and after the fill. That really works! Other than that, I went about my day after the fill, and even went to the gym. By nighttime, the discomfort was completely gone and I would forget all about it until my next appointment.   —Michelle

My doctor began filling my expanders with 120 cc every seven days. I was very uncomfortable for two or three days afterward. It felt like a metal band was crushing my ribs. I finally asked him to put in only 60 cc at a time. My expansion took longer, but it was more tolerable.   —Lin

Living in Limbo

After your initial reconstruction surgery, you'll leave the hospital with a surgical bra. When your doctor clears you to wear your own bra, be sure it fit wells and doesn't compress the expander. Avoid underwire bras, which can put too much pressure on the inframammary fold of your new breast, until your surgeon says you've healed sufficiently to wear them again.

Dressing during the expansion process can be a challenge. During unilateral expansion, your growing breast won't be the same size or shape as your healthy breast, so it may be difficult to find a bra that fits both. Early on in the process, a small prosthesis in your bra may help to correct an imbalance in your shape. As your breast mound grows larger, it may be higher and larger than your natural breast; camouflage is often the best strategy during this stage. Try going without a bra, or wear a comfy T-shirt topped with a dark shirt or sweater. Draw the eye away from your chest with diagonal stripes and asymmetrical prints. In cooler weather, try vests and scarves. You can also wear a padded mastectomy bra while your new breast is being expanded. As your breast mound grows, remove some of the stuffing from that side of the bra to give yourself a more symmetrical look.

Although you may feel as though the expansion process will never end, and you may become impatient with the cosmetic annoyances, there is light at the end of the tunnel. Don't be disheartened with your lumps, bumps, and dents. Hang in there if you feel lopsided or misshapen or if your reconstructed breast seems flatter or rounder than you expected. You may even experience "neck cleavage," where the expander rides high up on the chest, just beneath the collarbone. Don't be overly concerned with incisions that seem uneven or puckered; they can be improved during your *exchange surgery*. Remember, you're a work in progress. Expanders are temporary, your discomfort is temporary, and this isn't the way your finished reconstructed breast will look or feel. Keep the end result in mind, and in a few weeks your expansion will be complete.

Exchange Surgery

In three or four months, when your breast skin is adequately stretched and your expander reaches optimum fullness and is settled into the pocket, it's time to exchange the expander for your implant. You may need to wait a while longer if your surgeon wants to give your irradiated skin more time to heal or if your schedule causes a delay. Some women wait several months before swapping their expanders for implants.

Some expanders are adjustable, with an outer layer of silicone and an inner chamber that is inflated with saline. These combined expander-implants do double duty: saline can be added or removed to fine-tune your breast size during the six months after the implant is fully expanded. Then the fill port and tubing are removed, which triggers the expander to seal itself. The expander becomes the implant, eliminating the need for exchange surgery.

Exchange surgery is an outpatient procedure done under general anesthesia in a hospital or surgical facility. Once you're asleep, the surgeon reopens your mastectomy scar and removes the expander. He may also remove scar tissue from the pocket, which will soften the overall appearance of your breast. He then inserts your new implant into the pocket and, if necessary, adjusts the pocket so that your new breast is even with your opposite breast. If you're having bilateral reconstruction, the surgeon makes sure both breasts are evenly positioned. The incision is closed, and your chest is bound with a hospital dressing to discourage swelling.

Compared with your initial operation, exchange surgery is a snap. The procedure takes about an hour for each breast. You'll notice the difference as soon as you wake up: most if not all of the tightness will be gone, and your implants will feel vastly more comfortable than your expanders. You should be back to your normal routine in two or three days. In a few days, your surgeon will remove the hospital dressing, and for the first time, you'll get a look at your new breasts. They'll be a big improvement over the expanders, but they're still not the final product. Over the next few weeks, the swelling will subside and your implants will drop to a more normal position. They'll continue to settle and become softer over the next several months.

I was amazed to have hardly any swelling or bruising after my mastectomy, and I did have cleavage from the expanders! At first, they gave me a flat bulk, like a bodybuilder. My new breasts looked okay when I looked down, but there wasn't much there from a side view. I was so upset. Even though the expanders were better than no breasts at all; they were nothing like the breasts I had seen in my surgeon's patient photos. In hindsight, I should have listened to my surgeon, who said my implants would be very different. Of course, he was right. My implants are so much better than the expanders, and they continue to improve.   —Carole

Potential Problems

Most women don't have serious problems with tissue expanders, but complications can occur. Expanders aren't recommended if you have poor circulation in your chest, a history of poor wound healing, or an infection anywhere in your body. Delayed healing after mastectomy, insufficient blood flow to the skin, or other problems may also postpone or preclude using expanders for your reconstruction. Tobacco use, secondhand smoke, or other possible causes of blood flow problems may compromise circulation after mastectomy; if the breast skin dies, the expanders must be removed.

Expanding irradiated skin can be especially challenging and must proceed slowly (sometimes taking weeks longer than usual), especially when the skin is very thin or the tissue is scarred and thickened. Expanding the irradiated skin sometimes works and sometimes doesn't. It helps to have a plastic surgeon who has a good deal of experience working with irradiated skin and tissue.

Expanders can rupture if they're damaged or compressed excessively or if the port is defective. A ruptured expander leaks saline and loses volume and shape, and it needs to be removed to prevent infection. It's a frustrating setback, but a new expander can be put in and your reconstruction can then continue. Replacement may also be required when infection develops, an expander slips out of place, or significant capsular contracture occurs.

CHAPTER EIGHT

Tummy Tuck Flaps

Courage is being afraid but going on anyhow. —DAN RATHER

Not so long ago, the goal of breast reconstruction was simply to give a woman something more permanent than a prosthesis to fill her bra. *Tissue flap* reconstruction (also called *autologous reconstruction*) creates entirely new possibilities. A flap of your own skin and fat (and sometimes muscle) replaces breast tissue you've lost, recreating a soft breast that becomes an integral part of your body.

Tissue Flap Basics

All flap procedures move a segment of fat and skin, and sometimes muscle, up to the chest, where it is shaped into a breast. Flap reconstruction can be used as a primary method of recreating the breasts or used secondarily to replace failed implant reconstruction. (The opposite is also sometimes done: expanders or implants can replace a failed flap reconstruction.) Not all plastic surgeons perform autologous reconstruction, which requires special surgical skills. Compared with implant procedures, reconstruction with your own tissue is a longer operation and is initially more intense, but the start-to-finish interval is shorter than for traditional implant reconstruction with expansion (figure 8.1). As scars fade and tissue softens, the new breast improves over time. Flap surgery can be done only once from a particular *donor site*; if you need a future reconstruction, an implant or tissue flap from a different donor site must be used.

If you look at the human anatomy, you'll see three distinct tissue layers over the body's organs: skin on top, fat in the middle, and muscle underneath, with blood vessels running through all three layers. The distinction among the various tissue flap techniques, aside from the location of the donor site, is how these blood vessels are harvested. This is a critical part of flap reconstruction, because once in place in the chest, the transferred tissue needs a robust blood supply to survive. Surgeons use three types of flap procedures, each removing the needed blood vessels in a different way. Not all surgeons are qualified to do all procedures.

Attached (pedicled) flaps move a portion of skin, fat, and muscle under the skin to the chest. The blood supply is very reliable, because the entire flap remains attached by a strip of muscle to its original blood vessels at the donor site. The biggest drawback of an attached flap is that it sacrifices a perfectly healthy muscle, which isn't needed to build the breast but is taken only for the blood vessels that run through it.

Free flaps are complete transplants of tissue from the donor site to the chest. A free flap doesn't use all the muscle at the donor site; it includes just a portion that surrounds the necessary blood supply. A specially trained *microsurgeon* uses a high-powered magnifying lens and delicate instruments to reattach the tiny blood vessels in the flap to blood vessels in the chest—the sutures used are thinner than human hair. (A small piece of rib cartilage is sometimes removed to gain better access to the internal artery in the chest, particularly in women with narrow or small chests.) Because blood vessels are detached and reconnected at the mastectomy site, the supply of blood to the flap is temporarily interrupted. This isn't a problem if the reconnection is completed within 30 to 45 minutes.

Perforator flaps are the most advanced tissue transfers. Named for the small arteries that branch out and run through the muscle, these free flaps use only skin and fat, thereby preserving all of the muscle at the donor site.

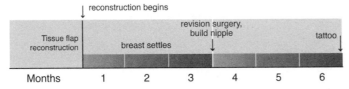

FIGURE 8.1. Tissue flap reconstruction timeline. Intervals may differ, depending on breast cancer treatment, preference of patient and surgeon, and complications that may delay completion.

The *perforator vessels* are carefully extracted from the underlying muscle and moved, along with the flap of skin and fat, to the mastectomy site, where they are reconnected to blood vessels in the chest. This requires the most microsurgical skill, experience, and technical savvy of all reconstruction procedures. Perforator flap reconstruction is complex and lengthy *microsurgery*, but compared with attached flap procedures, it's a less debilitating operation with a shorter hospital stay and quicker recovery, and it preserves muscle strength at the donor site.

ADVANTAGES OF TISSUE FLAP RECONSTRUCTION
- *It creates a breast with a natural feel, look, and movement.*
- *It offers a better chance of regaining sensation.*
- *No tissue expansion is required.*
- *It avoids the complications related to implants.*
- *It is less likely than implants to be compromised by radiation.*
- *Matching the normal droop of the opposite breast is easier (after unilateral mastectomy).*
- *It may improve contour at the donor site, especially hips and abdomen.*
- *It lasts a lifetime.*

DISADVANTAGES OF TISSUE FLAP RECONSTRUCTION
- *It scars an otherwise healthy part of the body.*
- *Some procedures sacrifice muscle.*
- *Surgery and recovery are longer and more intense than for implant procedures.*
- *It almost always requires a second-stage revision surgery.*
- *The area around the donor site incision may remain permanently numb.*
- *Future weight loss or gain may affect the volume of the new breast.*
- *Fewer surgeons are qualified and experienced in these techniques.*

Revision surgery. Once the breast has settled into its final position (at least three months after reconstruction), a return trip to the operating room for revision procedures can improve shape and symmetry. Fat liposuctioned through tiny incisions in your hips, thighs, or other locations can be injected into the new breast to fill sunken areas and improve contour. Scars can be revised and improved. These outpatient revision surgeries may last one, two, or three hours, depending on the amount of work to be done. Some surgeons focus primarily on the initial surgery; others consider revisions to be equally important to the completed reconstruction. Although not all problems can be fixed—there's only so much that can be done with radiation-treated tissue, for example—in the hands of a competent plastic surgeon, revision surgery can make subtle changes that improve the look of your new breasts. Your nipple(s) can be created at the same time.

Borrowing from the Abdomen

The abdomen is the most common donor site for flap reconstruction, providing a two-for-one benefit: the same tissue normally removed and discarded after a tummy tuck is used to create the breast. You come out of reconstructive surgery with new breasts *and* a flatter belly, thereby slimming your overall body contour. Abdominal tissue is a good choice for reconstruction because it has skin tone and texture similar to breast tissue.

Beneath the abdominal skin and fat are the rectus abdominis muscles, the long, flat "six-pack" muscles coveted by bodybuilders. You have two: one on the left and one on the right, both extending from the fifth, sixth, and seventh ribs to the pubic bone. These are the sit-up muscles that help you bend and flex at the waist and keep your abdominal organs in place. They have two primary sources of blood: the superior blood vessels at the top of the muscle near the rib cage and the deep inferior vessels at the bottom of the muscle near the groin. One or the other of these vessels are needed to nourish an abdominal tissue flap.

Abdominal flap procedures begin with a hip-to-hip elliptical incision between the navel and the pubic bone. The scar that remains will be covered by most bathing suits and underwear. Your belly button may look different after your surgery—during the operation, it's freed from the surrounding skin but remains attached to the abdominal wall. When the flap has been removed and the edges of the incision are pulled together, a new hole is made and the belly button is pulled through and sutured in place with tiny stitches.

Unless you have an abundance of excess abdominal tissue, you might wonder whether you should try to gain weight before your reconstruction, especially if you don't have enough abdominal tissue to make a breast of the size you'd like. Considering the health problems associated with obesity, it's probably inadvisable to recommend weight gain, particularly for someone who is already overweight. It all depends on your health and overall physical characteristics. Your surgeon may suggest you gain a few pounds if you're thin and a bit short of abdominal tissue to recreate your natural breast size: the more fat you have without affecting your health, the better the chance of completely replacing lost tissue.

Should You Gain Weight before Your Flap Surgery?
JOSHUA LEVINE, MD

Many patients ask whether or not they should gain weight prior to surgery to maximize the volume of the reconstructed breast. This is a logical question, because most of a tissue flap is made of fat, and it seems as though the more you weigh, the more fat will be available to use for breast reconstruction. The reality is not quite that simple. Overall, there is no benefit to gaining weight prior to autologous breast reconstruction, and there is the disadvantage of increasing your perioperative risk. Patients should be in top physical condition prior to surgery. The greater your level of fitness, the faster you will recover. So, it is difficult to advise a patient to gain weight, because of the obvious health and surgical risks of obesity. It is also extremely difficult to predict where someone will gain weight. Weight gain or loss is usually distributed throughout the body, and it is impossible to gain weight preferentially in the area that will be used for breast reconstruction. Thus there is an overall proportional change in the body, including the breasts. So if one were to gain or lose weight preoperatively, the breasts and donor area would grow or shrink together. Therefore the current breast size would be the same relative to the donor area, and the ultimate result would be exactly the same.

TRAM Flap Procedures

Introduced in the 1980s, the *transverse rectus abdominis myocutaneous (TRAM) flap* was the first abdominal flap technique developed for breast reconstruction. It was a significant step forward, because it gave women an alternative to implant reconstruction and an opportunity to have new breasts of their own living tissue. While *attached (pedicled) TRAM* isn't the most advanced flap reconstruction, it's still the most common, because it doesn't require microsurgical skill and it is widely available.

How an attached TRAM is done. A flap of skin, fat, and most of the underlying muscle is cut away from the lower abdomen and tunneled under the skin to the mastectomy site. Most of one rectus abdominis muscle is used to create a breast for unilateral reconstruction; both muscles are used for bilateral reconstruction. A strip of muscle remains tethered in place, acting as an umbilical cord between the flap and the original blood supply (figure 8.2). The upper portion of the flap is sutured into position to provide fullness at the top of the new breast, while the lower edge of the flap is folded under, shaped to match the

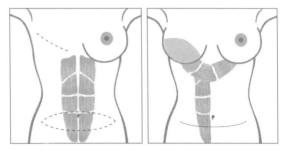

FIGURE 8.2. In the attached TRAM flap procedure, a flap of skin, fat, and muscle is tunneled under the skin to the chest but remains tethered by a strip of muscle to its blood supply in the abdomen.

size and contour of the opposite breast, and sutured in place. The edges of the abdominal incision are pulled together and closed.

Doing sit-ups and other abdominal exercises regularly for four to six weeks before your reconstruction will strengthen the muscles and increase blood flow to the donor site. To further improve the blood supply in the flap, some surgeons perform an outpatient "delay" procedure (not to be confused with delayed reconstruction) a week or two before the operation. The inferior blood vessels in the lower abdomen are divided to encourage the superior blood vessels in the upper abdomen—the ones that will supply the flap with blood—to grow stronger. This minor procedure involves two short incisions made along the same lines as the flap surgery, so you don't end up with additional scars.

Recovery. Attached TRAM surgery is serious business. You're recovering from not one, but two significant operations and the loss of one or both major abdominal muscles. It's the most difficult recovery of any breast reconstruction procedure (see table 8.1). You'll be immobile for the first few days, and for the first couple of weeks (or more, depending on your recovery) your movements will be limited. It will be difficult to stand straight, and you'll need help getting in and out of bed, especially if you've had a bilateral attached TRAM. While you're in bed or sitting, keeping your knees flexed will put less tension on your abdominal incision.

It's amazing how many movements involve the abdominal muscles—that's something you'll discover after a TRAM operation. Lifting, bending over, getting out of bed, and other movements we take for granted will be difficult until your incision heals. Initially, your abdomen will be sore and very tight; you'll feel a pulling sensation that may last for several months, but it slowly improves. It may take four to six weeks until you can begin gentle stretching; you'll gradually begin more vigorous movement and should be back to most routine activities within two months, although women sometimes require additional time to heal. You may feel tired for several more weeks as your energy level slowly returns. For the first two or three months after your surgery, your reconstructed breast will be swollen and look fuller than its final size. As the swelling subsides and the muscle thins from lack of exercise, your new breast will assume its final shape.

Most women have no long-term ill effects from an attached TRAM, other than an inability to do sit-ups. Some, however, find it difficult to get out of bed without using their arms. Removing the six-pack muscles and the *fascia* (the fibrous tissue covering the muscles) weakens the abdominal wall, which may limit some activities, particularly if you're athletic. You may need physical therapy to strengthen your remaining core muscles, and it may take six months or longer before you can return to golf, tennis, lifting weights, or other strenuous activities. A *hernia*, a bulge under the skin caused by the intestines poking through the muscle, may also occur as a result of the weakened abdominal wall. It's a painful condition that may require surgery to repair the muscle. The risk of hernia is greater if you're obese and less if your surgeon reinforces your abdomen with surgical mesh or an acellular dermal matrix during your reconstruction procedure. If you are planning to have this type of reconstruction, ask your surgeon how he will address the residual abdominal weakness. A different type of bulge may develop five or six months after the operation as a result of tunneling tissue under the skin; this usually recedes as the muscle atrophies and thins.

After an attached TRAM, it's questionable whether the abdominal walls are too weak to support a pregnancy without problems. There is little evidence or documented statistics one way or the other. However, there are reports of women who have had full-term pregnancies and delivered by cesarean section after an attached TRAM. If you hope to become pregnant one day, breast reconstruction with a muscle-sparing procedure or implants is probably a better choice.

When I woke up from my TRAM operation, I felt as though I had been hit by a bus. The first week or so, I thought I'd made a terrible mistake. I had medication and the pain improved a little each day, but the first week was awful. I couldn't stand or sit up straight for almost three weeks. —Teri

Honestly, my TRAM hurt like hell. I spent a lot of the day crying and just stayed on medication until I got better. Now I'm just as excited about my flat stomach as I am my new breast. For the first time in my life, I'm a babe! I'm wearing clothes I never would have worn before my surgery. —Monique

My cousin had a TRAM flap the year before I did. I was about 20 pounds overweight, she was in good shape. Her first seven or eight days were painful, and then she steadily improved. I had quite a bit of pain for three weeks. —Carrie

Variations on the TRAM flap. *Free TRAM* reconstruction uses the same tissue as the attached procedure, but removes a portion of the muscle that carries the blood supply. Instead of tunneling under the skin, the flap is freed from the donor site and transferred to the chest. Severing the blood vessels from the abdomen and reattaching them in the chest makes for a longer, more complex operation than an attached TRAM procedure, yet it does provide advantages: an improved blood supply that translates into less risk of necrosis or other healing problems. The more reliable blood supply is especially important in TRAM reconstruction involving obese women or those who smoke. Transplanting the flap to the mastectomy site, rather than tunneling it under the skin, also eliminates the bulges near the rib cage that often result from attached TRAM operations, and there is less risk of hernia. Although the muscle remains in the abdomen, it is cut across its width to remove the small amount that is included in the flap. So even though most of the muscle is left in place, much of the muscle function is destroyed. Recovery is similar to and may be a bit easier than what is experienced with an attached TRAM.

A *muscle-sparing TRAM* removes only a very small amount of muscle, often described as the size of a postage stamp. Because most of the muscle integrity and function at the donor site are preserved, you get the benefits of a free TRAM procedure without most of the disadvantages. Recovery is shorter and less painful, and the risk of hernia is reduced. Preserving most of the muscle retains abdominal function and strength, and surgical mesh isn't usually needed.

DIEP and SIEA Flaps

Why sacrifice a perfectly good muscle if you don't have to? That's the philosophy behind the *deep inferior epigastric perforator (DIEP) flap*, the most advanced method of breast reconstruction with abdominal tissue. DIEP flap reconstruction uses only what is needed for the new breast: the same fat and skin as an attached TRAM, but the blood vessels needed for the flap are removed from the donor muscle, instead of removing the muscle itself (figure 8.3). Overall complication rates are low, even among many patients who are active smokers or are obese.[1] You aren't

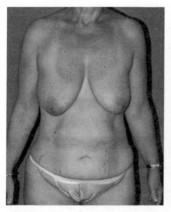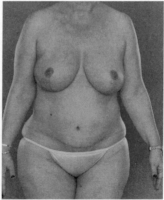

FIGURE 8.3. Before (*left*) and after (*right*) immediate bilateral DIEP reconstruction, with later nipple reconstruction and tattoos. *Images provided by Dr. Frank J. DellaCroce and The Center for Restorative Breast Surgery, LLC.*

a candidate for DIEP if you've already had a TRAM procedure or a full tummy tuck. A prior cesarean delivery, hysterectomy, tubal ligation, or gallbladder surgery doesn't usually eliminate DIEP as a possible reconstructive method, as long as you have enough tissue. Nor does previous liposuction or hernia repair necessarily preclude having DIEP, although a previous appendectomy may be a problem if it damaged the perforator blood vessels. The more abdominal surgeries you've had beforehand, the trickier it is to perform a DIEP with a successful outcome and the higher the risk of bulging or hernia.

How it's done. The flap of skin and fat is separated from the muscle and lifted up, exposing the inferior perforator arteries that branch out from a main artery and run through the muscle (figure 8.4). (A *periumbilical perforator [PUP] flap* uses the same tissue but includes a perforator artery that is closer to the navel.) An incision is then made in the muscle, and the blood vessels are carefully pulled out—it's important to preserve the adjacent motor nerves; if they're severed during the process, some abdominal muscle function could be lost. The flap is moved up to the mastectomy site, the blood supply is reconnected in the chest, and the tissue is shaped into a breast; the muscle stays fully functional in the abdomen. From the outside, there's little visible difference between a breast created with a TRAM or a DIEP. The difference, which is significant, is all on the inside. Few surgeons have the meticulous skill needed to perform this complex operation; even fewer perform it regularly.

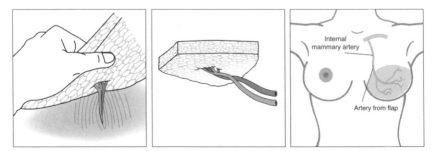

FIGURE 8.4. In perforator flap reconstruction, the flap is lifted (*left*), the perforator artery and veins are detached from the muscle (*center*), and these vessels are reconnected to blood vessels in the chest (*right*).

Variations on the DIEP flap. DIEP flap techniques can be modified for thin women who don't have quite enough abdominal tissue to rebuild their breasts. In an *extended DIEP*, the standard hip-to-hip incision is lengthened to include both abdominal and hip fat to provide additional volume. The *stacked DIEP* (also called a *double DIEP*) is an innovative solution that combines both sides of the abdomen to create a single breast; the entire abdominal flap is harvested in a single piece and folded over to create the breast, or both sides are harvested separately and stacked one on top of the other.[2] The result is a new breast that has more fullness and projection than a breast made from a single abdominal flap.

In a small percentage of women, the superficial inferior epigastric artery is the dominant blood supply to the abdomen (figure 8.5). Although the surgery and cosmetic result of a *superficial inferior epigastric artery (SIEA) flap* are essentially the same as those for a DIEP flap, SIEA blood vessels are found in the fatty tissue just beneath the skin and can be taken without cutting into the muscle at all. Recovery is improved, because the abdominal muscle is not only spared but undisturbed. A SIEA flap isn't possible for most women, for several reasons: the superficial blood vessels are usually too small to support the flap, or they've already been cut during a previous cesarean delivery or hysterectomy, or they don't exist.

Some flap reconstruction patients, usually those who have had other abdominal surgery, have perforator arteries that are damaged or too small to adequately supply the flap; in this case, a free TRAM can be performed instead. Mapping the blood vessels to determine the exact location and caliber of the blood flow before surgery saves time in the operating room. Blood vessels can be evaluated with a handheld pencil *Doppler* (a kind of powerful stethoscope that detects the sound of blood flow in perforators) during your consultation appointment or with color Doppler ultrasound, a special MRI, or a CT angiogram. Similar internal mapping can be performed in the operating room before an incision is made, by using a special dye and a

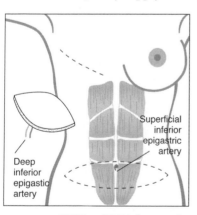

FIGURE 8.5. DIEP and SIEA flaps use fat and skin but no muscle.

technology called the SPY Imaging System to assess the perforator vessels as they travel through the tissue.

Finding a DIEP/SIEA surgeon. The most important factor in a perforator flap reconstruction, including DIEP and SIEA, is choosing a microsurgeon who routinely performs these procedures. Most reconstructive surgeons aren't trained in microsurgical breast reconstruction, but it is catching on. According to the American Society of Plastic Surgeons, more than 6,800 DIEP surgeries were performed in 2011, compared with just 1,900 in 2005. A physician's experience with DIEP reconstruction makes all the difference, and operating intervals and success rates vary among individual surgeons. Those who routinely perform DIEP reconstruction are likely to complete the procedure in less time than those who do not, and their success rates may be higher.

The only person qualified to assess whether you have enough tissue for a DIEP reconstruction is a plastic surgeon who routinely performs the procedure. If a surgeon who performs only TRAM or other non-DIEP procedures decides you don't have enough belly fat for a DIEP, an experienced DIEP surgeon may disagree. Likewise, if a surgeon says he needs to take only a small portion of muscle for a DIEP, he's actually talking about a free TRAM or muscle-sparing TRAM. You're lucky if you have an accomplished DIEP surgeon nearby (if you don't, check the list of microsurgeons at www.breastrecon .com). Most women must travel out of state for microsurgical reconstruction.

Recovery. Patients have less pain and get back to their normal activities sooner after DIEP than other abdominal flap procedures; it's still major surgery that requires recuperation (table 8.1). Being physically fit before your surgery will speed your recovery. It'll probably be at least 3 days before you can walk and another week or 10 days until you can stand upright and walk normally. Each day you'll feel progressively better and less fatigued. Many women return to work in about 4 weeks, while some require additional recovery. Strenuous exercise should be avoided for at least a couple of months after your surgery. By 6 weeks (and maybe sooner), you'll be able to drive and resume your routine activities. As for all surgeries, recovery varies from patient to patient.

TABLE 8.1. Intervals for abdominal flap reconstruction and recovery

Flap type	Surgery and hospital stay	Most routine activities resumed*
Attached TRAM	4–6 hours; 4–5 days in hospital	At 4–6 weeks
Free TRAM	6–8 hours; 4–5 days in hospital	At 4–6 weeks
DIEP or SIEA	6–8 hours; 3–5 days in hospital	At 2–4 weeks

Note: Reflects bilateral reconstruction without complications. Surgical expertise and individual healing affect recovery times.
*Additional time needed to regain full strength and mobility.

I play a lot of tennis, so I was in pretty good shape before my surgery. I wanted to get back on the court as soon as possible, so I had a DIEP operation. I was out of it for several days, although I recovered well and was back to most of my routine in about a month.   —Casey

When I decided to have DIEP reconstruction, I met with many surgeons. When my hometown doctors said I didn't have enough donor tissue, I traveled across most of the country for my surgeries and have never looked back—I returned home with two beautiful D-cup breasts. The experience was surreal but I chose the most competent and caring doctors I have ever met in my entire life. I now live in Israel and when my doctors here see my results, they are blown away. My recovery was uneventful; only some spitting stitches and hypertrophic scars. I was walking around by the third week and was [walking] up to four miles in another week or two. I drove by week six and returned to my desk job the following week. Five years later, I live a normal life. I see my scars but I do not regret my surgery one bit. —Debbie

Potential Problems

Although flap reconstruction with your own tissue doesn't involve the problems associated with breast implants, problems may occur. The success of a tissue flap reconstruction relies primarily on the strength of its blood supply. If the flap has adequate blood, it survives. If it doesn't, a portion of it may die off and become unusually firm; it can be removed or left as is. Or the entire flap may die and will need to be removed, but this isn't very common. An area of the new breast that appears much harder than the rest can also result from formation of scar tissue. This can often be remedied by routine massage and just the passage of time—in many instances, the tissue softens on its own in due time.

Other complications that may result from reconstruction surgery are discussed in chapter 15.

CHAPTER NINE

Other Flap Methods

Shoot for the moon. Even if you miss, you'll land among the stars. —LES BROWN, MOTIVATIONAL SPEAKER

If abdominal flap reconstruction isn't right for you, your breasts can be recreated with tissue from your back, buttocks, hips, or thighs. Although these procedures are used less often than implants or abdominal flaps, they produce very good reconstructive results.

The Latissimus Dorsi Flap

Originally developed to replace chest muscles after a radical mastectomy, *latissimus dorsi (lat) flap* reconstruction uses the large upper back muscle that runs from the shoulder to the hip. Many surgeons prefer to offer TRAM or DIEP procedures instead, but the lat flap is still a common method of reconstruction and an alternative if you're very thin and don't have enough donor tissue elsewhere. Depending where you live, it may be the only flap procedure available. Because the back has less fat than other donor sites, this method of reconstruction typically creates only a small to moderately sized breast and is most often combined with an implant (with or without tissue expansion). The donor site scar runs horizontally across the back and is easily covered by a bra. Some scars are diagonal and aren't as easily hidden, so if you choose this procedure for your reconstruction, talk to your surgeon about the placement of your incision.

A flap of fat and muscle from the back has a reliable blood supply and generally provides good results with few problems. For that reason, plastic surgeons frequently recommend this reconstructive method for breast cancer patients who have had radiation therapy. The flap brings healthy tissue to the chest and covers the implant completely, so rippling, wrinkling, and capsular contracture occur less often than with other implant

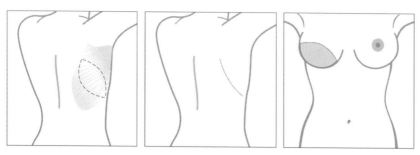

FIGURE 9.1. The latissimus dorsi flap is tunneled under the skin from the back to the chest (*left*), leaving a scar beneath the shoulder blade (*center*). An expander or implant is often added to increase volume (*right*).

procedures.[1] It isn't a preferred option if you have circulatory problems, persistent pain, or weakness in your back or shoulder. Other methods of reconstruction may be better if you've had previous surgery in or adjacent to the underarm (which can disrupt blood flow to the flap) or near your lungs or heart (which can affect blood supply to the back).

How it's done. This is an attached flap procedure. Once the mastectomy has been completed, you're turned to rest on your side or front. An ellipse of skin, fat, and part of the latissimus dorsi muscle is tunneled under the skin and across the armpit to the mastectomy site (figure 9.1). Once in place, the flap remains connected to its blood supply in the back. You're then returned to your back, and the flap is placed over the pectoralis muscle in the chest. If an expander or implant is used (as it most often is with this type of reconstruction), the latissimus muscle is sutured onto the lower edge of the pectoralis muscle, creating an instant pocket with overall coverage.

Recovery. Getting back to normal after a lat flap isn't as long or as painful as recovery after abdominal procedures, especially an attached TRAM operation. Your upper back may be sore for five or six weeks and will be numb for a few months until the nerves regenerate, and your underarm will be sore from tunneling the flap around to the chest. Any discomfort is usually controlled adequately with over-the-counter pain medication. The back is more prone to developing a *seroma* (a collection of fluid at the incision) than other donor sites, particularly if you're carrying a lot of extra weight, so you'll need surgical drains in your back and at your new breast for 10 to 14 days. You'll be restricted from stretching or overusing the donor site for a few weeks; you'll need six to eight weeks to regain full range of motion in your arm. It will be quite a bit longer before the tightness in your back begins to disappear; it may take at least three or four months before you can resume heavy lifting or return to strenuous activities (see table 9.1). Deep breathing and routinely stretching your back and shoulders will help you regain range of motion and mobility. Your doctor may recommend physical therapy to help you along. Taking the latissimus dorsi muscle doesn't cause significant weakness or interfere with routine activities for most women, because other muscles in the back compensate for the loss. You may notice reduced performance if you swim, golf, play tennis, cross-country ski, row, do pull-ups, or engage in other activities that depend heavily on shoulder or back strength. (If you stand facing a wall and push against it, the latissimus dorsi is the muscle that enables that movement.)

Potential problems. Back flap reconstruction generally has a low rate of complications compared with other flap procedures. If a problem develops, it's more likely to occur in your back than in your new breast. Necrosis of the flap tissue is rare, because the blood supply is very reliable. Bulges sometimes develop under the arm from tunneling the flap to the chest, similar to the bulges that may form after attached TRAM procedures. As the muscle atrophies over time, the bulge shrinks, although it may never disappear completely. Infections are uncommon, but if they occur, they're treated with antibiotics.

Variations on the lat flap. Some surgeons perform *endoscopic latissimus dorsi reconstruction*. This procedure transfers muscle entirely through the mastectomy incision or a small incision under the arm, leaving you with an unscarred back and a less painful recovery. Not many surgeons offer this technique, however. When the back (especially the lower back) has a generous excess of skin and fat, an *extended latissimus dorsi* procedure can be performed to transfer a larger flap to the breast, eliminating the need for an implant. This procedure combines the standard lat flap with fatty tissue from the lower back, so it leaves a longer scar. The length of the operation and recovery time are about the same as for a traditional lat flap. Obese women are at higher risk for post-op complications after this reconstruction.

During a *muscle-sparing latissimus dorsi* procedure, an incision is made lower on the back and the muscle is divided vertically: a small portion is used to create the breast, while the rest remains functional in the back. Patients have good cosmetic results, retain shoulder strength, and experience little or no seroma afterward.[2] Because the muscle is spared, recovery is less painful and somewhat quicker than for traditional latissimus dorsi reconstruction—most patients spend just one night in the hospital.

The *thoracodorsal artery perforator (TAP or TDAP) flap* is a muscle-sparing perforator version of the lat flap that is rotated to the chest. It doesn't typically yield enough tissue for full breast reconstruction and is usually limited to correcting post-lumpectomy defects or improving the contour and volume of other reconstruction procedures. The *intercostal artery perforator (ICAP) flap* takes a small amount of tissue from under the arm, beside the breast. It is also used to partially reconstruct breasts after lumpectomy and is rarely used to recreate full breasts after mastectomy.

ADVANTAGES OF THE BACK FLAP
- *The procedure is widely available.*
- *It provides a reliable method of reconstruction.*
- *It doesn't restrict or weaken most normal movement after recovery.*
- *Recovery is shorter and less painful than for abdominal flaps.*
- *There's less chance of capsular contracture when used with an implant.*

DISADVANTAGES OF THE BACK FLAP
- *It usually requires an implant for a moderately sized breast.*
- *It leaves a long scar down the back (unless endoscopic surgery is performed).*
- *The flap skin may have different color and texture than the rest of the breast.*
- *You may require physical therapy to regain strength and range of motion.*
- *This type of reconstruction may restrict certain movements.*

I'm the world's biggest chicken when it comes to pain. I asked my doctor what method of reconstruction was the least painful. He recommended using the muscle in my back and a small implant. My recovery wasn't bad and my new breast is fine.   *—Marta*

As an aerobics instructor, I didn't want to risk reduced abdominal strength, even though my doctor said I'd be okay after TRAM reconstruction. I read about the back flap in a magazine. I'm glad I did, because my surgery went very well.   *—Dee Dee*

GAP Flaps

Posterior, derriere, backside, rump, tush, gluteus maximus. Popular jargon aside, a well-padded bottom can be a prime source for breast reconstruction. The tissue that provides a *gluteal artery perforator (GAP) flap* has a high fat-to-skin ratio and a robust blood supply, producing excellent reconstructive results without needing the muscle. Buttock fat is firm; it forms soft breasts with good volume and projection. You probably have enough gluteal tissue to recreate one or both breasts, even if you're slender and

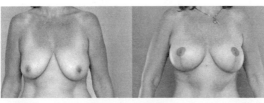
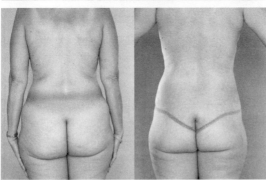

lack sufficient abdominal fat for DIEP or TRAM. You may not be a candidate for this type of reconstruction if you've already had gluteal liposuction.

Except for the donor site location, the *superior gluteal artery perforator (SGAP)* procedure is similar to the DIEP technique. A slanted elliptical incision is made on the upper buttock, from the outer hip to the intergluteal cleft between the cheeks—the resulting scar is prominent across the top of the buttock, although it falls below the panty line (figure 9.2). A flap of skin and fat is carefully re-

FIGURE 9.2. Before (*left*) and after (*right*) immediate bilateral GAP reconstruction, followed by nipple reconstruction and tattoos. *Images provided by Dr. Frank J. DellaCroce and The Center for Restorative Breast Surgery, LLC.*

moved where the upper buttock meets the hip—excess fat in the "love handles," the fatty area just below the waist, or in the lower back can also be incorporated into the flap if extra tissue is required—and the gluteal artery feeding the tissue is separated from the muscle. The flap is then reattached to the chest and shaped into a breast.

The less common *inferior gluteal artery perforator (IGAP)* procedure removes a flap from the lower part of the buttock through an incision in the crease (figure 9.3). The surgeon must take care to protect the sciatic nerve while dissecting the blood vessels; nicking it can cause irreparable sciatic damage. This is less likely in the

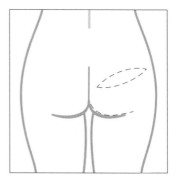

FIGURE 9.3. SGAP reconstruction uses a diagonal elliptical flap from the upper part of the buttock. IGAP reconstruction uses a flap that follows the natural crease beneath the buttock.

hands of experienced IGAP surgeons. The in-the-crease flap uses excess fat low on the buttock to create new breasts. The scar is hidden in the crease beneath your bottom, but the procedure tends to square off the natural curve of the lower buttock, which can result in a somewhat flattened, more masculine-looking derriere.

Borrowing gluteal tissue doesn't permanently impair strength or functional movement; it does flatten the buttock, particularly after an SGAP procedure. If your surgeon removes the fascia covering the gluteus maximus muscle, the bulk of the muscle falls into the space created by the flap removal, often preserving the natural contour.[3] Symmetry can be restored during revision surgery by lifting the opposite buttock or rounding out the donor site with fat liposuctioned from your hips or thighs.

How it's done. GAP flap surgery is a lengthy and meticulous operation, requiring several hours under anesthesia. You must be turned twice during the procedure. When it's performed as an immediate reconstruction, you are first positioned on your back. Once the mastectomy is completed, you're gently turned onto your front so the surgeon can harvest fat and skin from your backside. You're then returned to your back to complete the reconstruction. Delayed GAP flap reconstruction is similar yet shorter, since the mastectomy has already been done. Like abdominal flaps, GAP flap surgery comes with a bonus of its own: a higher firmer buttock, similar to a buttock lift, resulting from pulling the skin together when the incision is closed.

Few surgeons perform gluteal perforator flaps, and even fewer perform both sides simultaneously. Most GAP surgeons limit this operation to one breast at a time, requiring two separate 10- to 12-hour operations a few months apart to accomplish bilateral reconstruction—that means two surgeries, two bouts with the effects of anesthesia, two recoveries, and a very long overall reconstruction timeline (see table 9.1). If you're interested in this bilateral procedure, you might want to consider experienced GAP flap surgeons who reconstruct both breasts in a single operation (consult the list at www.breastrecon.com), which usually takes 8 to 10 hours. One surgeon harvests a flap and rebuilds a breast on one side, while a second surgeon does the same thing on the opposite side.

> When my implants failed, my only other option was a gluteal flap; I didn't have enough fat in my stomach. Though I didn't look forward to another surgery and recovery, I was pleasantly surprised after my GAP. I was tired for several days, but I had far less discomfort than I did when I had tissue expanders.   —Kat

> The best thing about the gluteal scar is that I don't have to see it every time I look in the mirror.   —Sondra

Recovery. Recuperating from GAP reconstruction is generally less painful and quicker than recovery from TRAM or DIEP reconstruction. You'll feel a dull ache in the area around the gluteal incisions; that shouldn't keep you from being out of bed for a short walk the day after your GAP surgery. Surgical drains at the chest usually remain for about a week; the drains at your hip may be required for two or three weeks. Wearing a compression bra around the clock for two weeks and a surgical compression girdle for two to four weeks helps to prevent seroma and reduces post-op pain by supporting the incision. It may be difficult to sit comfortably or lie on your back; most GAP patients discover which positions are more comfortable until healing occurs, and until the nerves surrounding the incision regenerate, the area will be numb. If you have an IGAP procedure, the back of your thigh may also be numb for quite some time until you regain feeling.

ADVANTAGES OF THE GLUTEAL FLAP

- *There is no loss of muscle function.*
- *The failure rate is low when performed by a skilled and experienced microsurgeon.*
- *The donor scar is usually hidden by swimsuits and underwear.*
- *Even thin women usually have enough buttock tissue for reconstruction.*
- *It produces a firmer breast than tissue from other donor sites.*
- *The recovery is less painful than for abdominal flap surgery.*

DISADVANTAGES OF THE GLUTEAL FLAP

- *The operation is lengthy and complex.*
- *Few surgeons perform GAP flap surgery.*
- *Even fewer surgeons offer simultaneous bilateral GAP flap surgery.*
- *There's a risk of sciatica if the nerve is damaged (particularly during IGAP).*
- *A unilateral flap causes buttock asymmetry.*

Using Fat from the Thighs

The abdomen and buttocks aren't the only sources for tissue flap reconstruction. Many microsurgeons offer flap reconstruction that uses tissue from the thighs and hips.

If you want small to moderate breasts and you carry more weight in your thighs than in your abdomen, a *transverse upper gracilis (TUG) flap* may be a good reconstructive option. Thigh tissue is soft and pliable, the blood supply to the flap is reliable, and losing the gracilis muscle doesn't affect form or function. TUG surgery is less complex than DIEP or GAP procedures, and it isn't necessary to turn you during the operation.

How it's done. An incision is made high on the thigh, just under the groin crease on the front of the leg, through which a crescent of fat and muscle is removed. The TUG flap is a free flap; it removes part of the muscle surrounding the blood vessels, requiring microsurgical skills to reattach the vessels to the blood supply in the chest. A TUG flap incision is generally well hidden just below the groin crease, and most women don't have a noticeable indentation where the flap was removed. The TUG flap also provides a

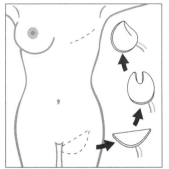
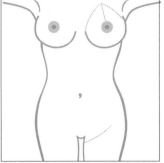

FIGURE 9.4. The TUG flap uses tissue from the thigh; the flap is folded over (*left*) and moved to the chest (*right*).

unique advantage over other flap types: folding the crescent shape creates an almost perfect cone, providing excellent projection and facilitating nipple reconstruction during the initial procedure (figure 9.4), though many surgeons prefer to create the nipple three or four months later, during revision surgery. A less common variation of the TUG flap, the *transverse upper thigh (TUT) flap*, uses a different blood supply and spares the muscle.

The TUG procedure is similar to an inner thigh lift. If you carry considerable weight at the donor site, you'll have new breasts and thinner thighs. When the procedure is combined with liposuction along your outer thighs during revision surgery, you may come out of your breast surgery with a vastly slimmed down body contour. Unlike abdominal flaps, a TUG procedure is possible even if your thighs have previously been liposuctioned.[4]

TUG Flap with Immediate Nipple Reconstruction

R. BUNTIC, MD

The inner thigh skin and fat of the TUG flap can provide superior aesthetic results compared with other microsurgical options. The generous size of the skin island that can be harvested with the gracilis muscle allows for shaping the flap in a cone-like fashion, more closely resembling natural breast anatomy than the relatively flat skin of a DIEP, SIEA, or GAP flap. The dog ear at the central portion of the folded TUG flap recreates nipple projection; the resulting nipple-areola is aesthetically superior to those reconstructed with local flaps or skin grafts. The characteristics and skin color of the flap do not require tattooing or local flaps. Inner thigh skin is slightly darker than skin on the chest, and when contracted and allowed to pucker slightly it becomes even darker. This color difference in the breast skin also allows for a more natural-looking areola than one that is simulated by tattooing. And unlike the rectus muscle in the abdomen, the gracilis muscle is entirely expendable and has no potential to form a hernia. There is a trade-off: a visible scar that remains on the inner thigh.

Recovery. Compared with recovery from an abdominal flap reconstruction, recuperating from TUG flap surgery is quicker and less painful, yet more awkward, because of the incision placement. You'll walk the day after your surgery; however, you'll need to minimize movements that flex your hips or spread your legs for the next couple of weeks, to avoid putting tension on the thigh incision. Too much thigh movement may delay healing—this doesn't dramatically affect your final outcome, though it may affect how the incision heals; eventually, *scar revision* may be needed to achieve an acceptable result. You'll be sore for about a week or two, and then you'll begin to improve each day (table 9.1).

ADVANTAGES OF THE TUG FLAP
- *The flap has a reliable blood supply.*
- *The procedure provides an inner thigh lift.*
- *There's a minimal risk of complications.*
- *There's no noticeable loss of muscle function.*

DISADVANTAGES OF THE TUG FLAP
- *The amount of available tissue may be sufficient for only a small to moderately sized breast.*
- *The scar may be visible, depending on where the incision is made on the thigh.*
- *Recovery may be a bit awkward.*

TABLE 9.1. Intervals for other flap reconstructions and recovery

Flap type	Surgery and hospital stay	Most routine activities resumed[*]
Lat flap	4–6 hours; 3–4 days in hospital	At 3–6 weeks
GAP flap	8–10 hours;[†] 3–4 days in hospital	At 4–6 weeks
TUG flap	6–8 hours; 3–4 days in hospital	At 4–6 weeks

Note: Reflects bilateral reconstruction without complications. Surgical expertise and individual healing affect recovery times.
[*]Additional time needed to regain full strength and mobility.
[†]Procedure performed by an experienced two-surgeon team.

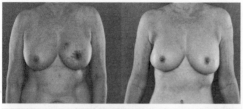

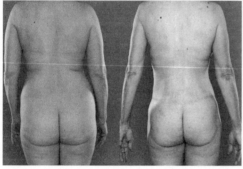

FIGURE 9.5. Before (*left*) and after (*right*) immediate bilateral reconstruction with combined DIEP and hip flaps. *Images provided by Dr. Frank J. DellaCroce and The Center for Restorative Breast Surgery, LLC.*

Variations on thigh flaps. Tissue can be taken from any part of the thigh, although aside from the TUG flap, most flaps from this area are not cosmetically advantageous, considering the very visible scars. The *lateral transverse thigh flap*, also called the *Reubens flap*, uses tissue from the upper outer thigh. This free flap operation is rarely performed, because it disfigures the contour of the thigh and leaves a long, obvious scar. A unilateral flap with this method causes very visible asymmetry with the opposite leg. The *anterolateral perforator flap* is popular for repairing head and neck injuries, and some plastic surgeons use it as a source for breast reconstruction. While it's easily accessed and has a good blood supply, it's used infrequently to recreate breasts, because it takes tissue from the front of the thigh and leaves very visible scarring. The *profunda artery perforator (PAP) flap* uses the fatty part of the upper thigh below the buttock. It's a newer alternative to GAP reconstruction, that leaves the patient with an acceptable overall contour, doesn't require repositioning during surgery, and creates a scar that is well hidden in the buttock crease.

Using Fat from the Hips

The *lumbar artery perforator (LAP) flap* is a variation of the SGAP procedure. It uses the "love handles" to reconstruct the breasts. Removing tissue in this area slims the hips and also lifts the buttock. It leaves a horizontal scar where the waist meets the upper buttock that is usually hidden by most bathing suits or underwear. LAP reconstruction preserves muscle, so recovery is shortened and less uncomfortable than for other procedures that sacrifice muscle. Hip flaps can be combined with other flap procedures (see figure 9.5).

CHAPTER TEN

Altering the Opposite Breast

Being happy doesn't mean everything's perfect; it just means you've decided to see beyond the imperfections.

—UNKNOWN

When a plastic surgeon recreates both breasts at the same time, he or she can usually ensure they're of similar size, shape, and position, with nicely centered nipples. Unilateral reconstruction presents a different problem: how to achieve balance between the reconstructed breast and your natural breast. An optional cosmetic procedure on your natural breast can help you obtain the best possible symmetry. Your reconstructed breast may not be an exact match, but even natural breasts aren't identical. Often, however, reconstructing one breast and altering the other minimizes differences. This opportunity for a breast makeover is something many women may have long considered yet never pursued. (Health insurance companies that cover mastectomy are required by the Women's Health and Cancer Rights Act to pay for modifications to the remaining breast to achieve symmetry, as part of your overall reconstruction.)

If you're having unilateral mastectomy, you have three alternatives for your opposite breast:

- Leave it as it is. If you prefer not to alter your remaining breast, symmetry with your reconstructed breast will depend on the reconstruction method you choose. A flap reconstruction offers a better chance of matching your natural breast, because the living tissue can be sculpted and shaped to better match the shape and natural droop, but an implant cannot.
- Surgically modify it. Your healthy breast can be reduced, lifted, or enlarged with an implant to match your reconstructed breast.
- Remove and reconstruct it. If you have a high risk for contralateral

breast cancer, you may want to consider prophylactic removal of your healthy breast. In that case, you'll have bilateral mastectomy and immediate reconstruction.

If you decide to have a little work done on your natural breast, ask to see your surgeon's before-and-after photos of reconstruction patients who have had the same cosmetic procedure you're considering. Notice how closely (or not) their reconstructed and modified breasts match. Ask the surgeon to explain the best and worst results you can expect. Discuss with her your preferences regarding breast size, how you would like your breast to look, how your nipples will be affected, and options for incision placement.

Breast Augmentation

Augmentation mammoplasty, which enlarges your breast by a full cup size or more, is the most common cosmetic procedure in the United States. Adding an implant will make your breast fuller and firmer.

How it's done. Breast augmentation is a relatively simple operation, performed while you're under general or local anesthetic. Implants are inserted through an incision made under the breast, around the bottom of the areola, or in the underarm—the underarm procedure makes for a more difficult surgery and leaves a scar that will show when you raise your arm (figure 10.1). Alternatively, some surgeons use a *transumbilical breast*

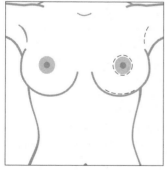

FIGURE 10.1. In breast augmentation, incisions are made around the bottom of the areola, under the breast, or in the underarm.

augmentation (TUBA) incision around the belly button, then tunnel the implant up through the fat under the skin to the chest. Although a TUBA incision leaves no scar on the breast, it's more difficult to reshape breast tissue after the implant is in place. If you'd like to consider a TUBA procedure, look for a surgeon who has experience doing this type of augmentation. For an augmentation procedure of any kind, you'll need a baseline mammogram before the procedure, and you'll need to have all future mammograms of that breast evaluated by specially trained radiology technicians.

Augmentation surgery is similar to the pocket procedure used for implant reconstruction. An implant is placed directly into a pocket created behind the chest muscle—there's no need for expansion. (Implants used for augmentation are often placed in front of the muscle, but positioning the implant under the muscle will better match your reconstructed breast.) Your newly augmented breast is positioned to match your reconstructed breast, and the incision is stitched closed and covered with a surgical compression bandage or a surgical bra.

Recovery. After surgery, your chest will feel heavy for several days. It may be bruised, swollen, and sore for two to four weeks. Cold compresses or ice packs will help reduce the swelling. Be patient if your breast is too high and excessively firm; it will drop and soften over the next several weeks as your skin and muscle stretch to accommodate the implant. You may feel tingling, burning, or sharp pains for a few weeks, and your nipple may be quite sensitive; even rubbing against clothing may make it itch or ache. Covering it with a small round Band-Aid until the sensitivity disappears will help. Most women can shower and return to restricted activities and work without heavy lifting within a week, although some require a few more days to recover. In three to four weeks you should regain normal range of motion and resume your routine activities. After six to eight weeks, the swelling subsides.

Potential problems. Aside from the possible risks inherent in surgery and implants, breast augmentation usually causes few problems. Less than 2 percent of women who have augmentation permanently lose some or all feeling in their nipple and areola and sometimes throughout the breast. If you have breastfed within a year prior to augmentation, you may spontaneously produce a milky discharge for several days after your operation; it's a condition called *galactorrhea* that usually stops on its own. Call your surgeon if your nipple discharges fluid that is yellow or green or has an odd smell. These are signs of infection and you may need antibiotics. If you have augmentation with a silicone implant and plan to breastfeed in the future, you may be concerned about the potential of passing silicone to your baby through breast milk. According to the American Academy of Pediatrics (www.aap.org), "It is unlikely that elemental silicon causes difficulty, because silicon is present in higher concentrations in cow's milk and formula than in milk of humans with implants."

Breast Reduction

If you're bothered by rashes, breathing problems, back pain, or other complications from breasts that are too big, *breast reduction (reduction mammoplasty)* can make life a lot more comfortable and boost your self-image. The size of your reduced breast and areola will be similar to your reconstructed breast and have overall better proportion to your body.

   How it's done. Breast reduction is a more complex procedure than augmentation and involves more downtime. It can be done in different ways, depending on your surgeon's preferred technique and how much tissue needs to be removed. You may have a lollipop incision—around the areola and down from the nipple to the bottom of the breast—or an anchor incision, a lollipop with an additional incision along the crease (figure 10.2). Alternatively, your surgeon may use a circular incision beyond the edges of the areola. The breast is then opened along the incision lines and excess tissue and skin are removed. When the amount of tissue to be eliminated is small, a less invasive incision can be made across the top of the areola or around it, or liposuction may be adequate.

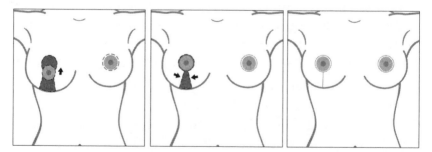

FIGURE 10.2. In breast reduction, excess fat and skin are removed through an anchor incision, and the nipple is repositioned higher on the breast (*left*). The edges of the incision are pulled together (*center*). The newly reduced breast closely matches the reconstructed breast (*right*).

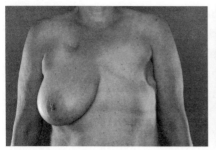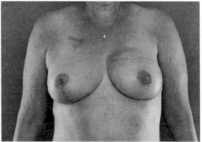

FIGURE 10.3. Before (*left*) and after (*right*) delayed DIEP flap reconstruction and reduction of the opposite breast for symmetry. *Images provided by Dr. Frank J. DellaCroce and The Center for Restorative Breast Surgery, LLC.*

During the operation, the nipple usually remains attached to its nerves and blood vessels on an island of skin that is pulled up and out of the way until excess tissue is removed. If the breasts are large, it may be necessary to completely remove the nipple and graft it to a higher position; this may cause permanent loss of feeling in the nipple. Once the excess tissue is removed, the nipple is recentered on the breast (figure 10.3). (If your areola is too large for your now smaller breast, it, too, can be reduced.) Both sides of the incision are pulled together, creating a firmer, tighter contour. A surgical drain is placed at the site, and the newly reduced breast is wrapped in an elastic bandage or a surgical compression bra.

Recovery. Breast reduction is a significant procedure and recovery can be uncomfortable. Any bruising, soreness, and swelling are routine side effects of reduction that dissipate as you heal. Most pain occurs in the first three or four days after surgery. After that, you'll be up and around, but restricted from lifting or exerting too much. Until you heal further, it may be painful to cough or sneeze. In about two weeks, your stitches will come out and you may return to work—your scars will be pink for six months or more. Most women are back to full activities in three to four weeks. Your plastic surgeon will remove your bandages a few days after your operation, although you'll need to wear a sports bra, surgical bra, or other compression garment around the clock for several weeks to support your breast as it heals. Initially, you can expect to lose some feeling in your nipples and breast skin; the feeling will return as your swelling subsides, although some women don't regain feeling for many months. Sensation returns gradually—you may have random shooting pains for several weeks, and your nipple and breast may be numb for several weeks or even up to a year. It may be 6 to 12 months before your breast settles into its new shape. It may swell and hurt when you have your first menstruation after reduction surgery. If you gain weight after your surgery, your reduced breast may regain some or all of its previous size.

Potential problems. Sensitivity in your breast will be reduced as a result of disturbing the nerves during surgery. Feeling returns over several weeks; a small percentage of women lose some or all feeling in their nipples. In very rare cases, the nipple and areola may die from loss of blood. If this occurs, a skin graft is required to rebuild the nipple. Your ability to breast-feed is more likely to be preserved when the nipple remains attached to the skin and the milk ducts are left intact. The likelihood of the ducts being damaged or severed increases if your nipple is removed from your breast during surgery or if your reduction involves a lot of tissue. If you're concerned about the ability to breastfeed in the future, discuss the procedure with your surgeon. The Breastfeeding After Breast and Nipple Surgeries website (www.bfar.org) provides information and support to mothers who want to breastfeed after reduction surgery or who have other breast or nipple procedures.

Breast Lift

All natural breasts head south over time. As gravity takes its toll, tissue loses elasticity, breasts hang lower on the chest, and areolae become larger. A *breast lift (mastopexy)* raises and reshapes a breast that sags because of age, excessive weight, pregnancy, hormones, or genetics. If your nipple points downward, a breast lift will reposition it so that it matches the nipple on your reconstructed breast. A breast lift doesn't reduce or enlarge the breast. However, the lift procedure can be combined with an augmentation or a reduction to achieve either result. Small sagging breasts can be lifted and augmented; overly large breasts can be lifted and reduced.

How it's done. Different incisions can be used, depending on the amount of skin to be removed, the position of your nipple and areola, and how

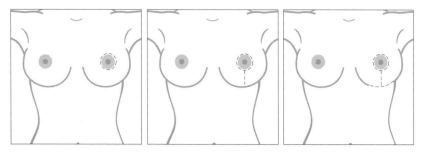

FIGURE 10.4. A breast lift is performed with periareolar (*left*), lollipop (*center*), or anchor (*right*) incisions.

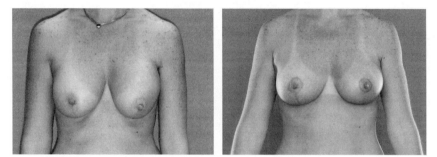

FIGURE 10.5. Before (*left*) and after (*right*) immediate stacked DIEP flap reconstruction of the left breast and lift of the opposite breast. *Images provided by Dr. Frank J. DellaCroce and The Center for Restorative Breast Surgery, LLC.*

much your breast sags (figure 10.4). If your breast is small with minimal sagging, a small segment of skin can be removed with an incision across the top of the areola or around it; the scars will be hidden in the border of the areola. A lollipop incision is often used to lift and reshape a moderately sagging breast, while a very large or heavily sagging breast may require an anchor incision. Once the incisions are made, the breast tissue is tightened and reshaped, and the nipple and areola are appropriately repositioned. Excess skin is removed, and the edges of the incision are sutured together. The same amount of breast tissue is now held together by less skin, so your breast is firmer and sits higher on your chest (figure 10.5). Some or all of your nipple sensation may be temporarily lost, but you can expect it to return as your breast heals.

Recovery. Your breast will be bruised for a few days and may be swollen for up to six weeks or more. You'll progress to a soft support bra within 7 to

TABLE 10.1. Intervals for breast modification procedures and recovery

Procedure	Surgery and hospital stay	Back to daily activities	Back to strenuous activities
Augmentation	1–2 hours; outpatient	1 week	3–4 weeks
Reduction	2–3 hours; outpatient	2–3 weeks	6–8 weeks
Lift	2–3 hours; outpatient	1 week	3–4 weeks

10 days; you mustn't lift anything over five pounds during this time or until your surgeon says it's okay to do so. For the next few weeks, you'll need to wear an athletic bra (no underwires) around the clock. As with other breast surgeries, you should refrain from activities or movements that strain your incisions, and you'll need to avoid sleeping on your front for at least three to four weeks. Most women can return to work within two weeks and resume full activities in three weeks (table 10.1).

Potential problems. Your nipple and breast may be numb for six weeks or more or until the swelling subsides. Until the swelling disappears, your nipples may be off-center or positioned unevenly, and minor revision surgery may be required to improve symmetry. Numbness may persist for up to a year and, in rare cases, may be permanent. A breast lift shouldn't affect your ability to breastfeed, because the milk ducts generally aren't disturbed. Breast lifts aren't permanent. Eventually, gravity, age, or other factors will cause them to sag again.

CHAPTER ELEVEN

Final Touches

Creating Your Nipple and Areola

> *There are only two ways to live your life. One is as though nothing is a miracle. The other is as though everything is a miracle.* —ALBERT EINSTEIN

You've made it through mastectomy. You have a new breast mound (or two), and unless you had a nipple-sparing mastectomy, you're now ready for the final reconstructive steps: creating new nipples and areolae. Nipple reconstruction is simple and minimally invasive. It does involve a bit more surgery, but it's minor compared with what you've been through thus far. You're in the reconstructive home stretch.

Icing on the Cake

Recreating your nipples is a physical and psychological milestone. *Nipple reconstruction* completes the restoration of your missing breast or breasts and, for many women, represents the end of the breast cancer experience. Creating a nipple is the icing on the reconstruction cake, although not everyone wants icing. You may consider your new breasts to be incomplete without nipples, or you may feel as though you just can't face another procedure and decide to skip nipple surgery altogether. After mastectomy and reconstruction, some women feel they need a break from surgery, and they wait for a year or longer before having their nipples created.

Perhaps you're concerned about the physical limitations of reconstructed nipples: they'll be permanent bumps on your breast mound that won't react to cold or touch, and they won't change from flat to erect and back to flat again, as natural nipples do, because they'll lack the infrastructure of nerves and small muscles to make that happen. If you have unilateral reconstruction, your new nipple will be standing at attention when your natural nipple isn't. With bilateral reconstruction, both nipples will always be raised, though they shrink considerably over time as they heal. This is something to keep in mind when you're deciding how small or how large you'd like your nipples to be.

Planning your procedure. New nipples can be created during revision surgery while you're under general anesthesia or anytime thereafter in a separate outpatient procedure under local anesthesia. (Your insurance company may consider an in-office nipple procedure as cosmetic and may cover related costs only when the nipple is created in a hospital or surgical facility.) Each nipple is formed in about an hour.

Before your plastic surgeon rebuilds your nipples, discuss how you would like them to look: As large as your natural nipples? Bigger? Smaller? Nipples can be made in numerous ways. Ask about your surgeon's preferred method and look at his before-and-after photos. If you're having unilateral reconstruction, let him know if you'd like your new nipple to be slightly off-center to match the nipple of your natural breast or precisely centered. If you've had bilateral reconstruction, your new nipples will be centered at the point of most projection on your breasts. Also consider how much projection you would like to have. Do you want the new nipples to be almost flat? Barely there? Initially, reconstructed nipples are prominent on the breasts, but eventually they flatten. If you prefer protruding nipples, your surgeon can augment them with fat, an acellular dermal matrix, or other implantable material. If you have microsurgical flap reconstruction, during that procedure your surgeon will remove a bit of cartilage to gain better access to arteries in the chest. Cartilage that is usually discarded can be banked under the skin during mastectomy and retrieved later and inserted into your recreated nipples. Discuss this with your surgeon before your flap reconstruction.

Questions for your plastic surgeon:

- How will you create my nipples and areolae?
- How many of these procedures have you done?
- Where will the procedure be performed and how long will it take?
- Will I need an anesthetic?
- Will I have any downtime from the procedure?

- How closely will my new nipple and areola match my healthy breast?
- Where will I have scars and how conspicuous will they be?
- Who will tattoo my nipples and areolae? What is his or her experience?
- What if I'm not satisfied with the location, color, or size?

My surgeon tried to convince me to "finish the job," but nipples didn't seem important. That was four years ago and I still don't regret my decision. If I change my mind, I can always have them added.   —*Karola*

Building the Nipple

These days, most surgeons fashion nipples from a small flap of breast skin. There are many ways to do this, and each surgeon has a preferred method. Most common are the skate and star flaps (figure 11.1). Other techniques include the bell flap, fishtail flap, omega flap, and numerous others, all named for the shape of the incision.

How it's done. To begin, the flap pattern is first marked on the breast. The surgeon makes incisions along the markings, freeing small flaps of skin from the breast and leaving a nipple-shaped nodule of fat protruding in the center. He then twists the ends of the skin flaps around and over that bump and stitches them closed. Antibiotic ointment and petroleum jelly are applied to protect the new nipples, which are then covered with protective bandages, with the nipple protruding through a hole cut in the center. Alternatively,

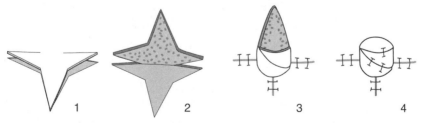

FIGURE 11.1. In nipple reconstruction, a star flap is created by excising and lifting breast skin along three sides of a star shape (1, 2). The two lateral points are wrapped around the top (3), which is tucked down and sutured in place (4).

your surgeon may cover the new nipples with a plastic protector or recommend that you use a maternity shield. No surgical drains are required.

Before mini-flaps were used to rebuild nipples, skin grafts were the preferred method. The surgeon transferred a circular patch of darkly pigmented skin from the labia or inner thigh to create the areola. Skin grafts are still useful to repair burns or wound defects, but they're really not necessary for nipple reconstruction. Nevertheless, some surgeons still prefer to use grafts, so it's worth asking about how your nipples will be created before you have the procedure done. The grafting process creates an additional scar, and the donor site remains sore for a week or two. There's a potential cosmetic issue too: if the skin graft has hair follicles, the new nipple may sprout hair. Another infrequent technique, called *nipple sharing*, uses a portion of a woman's healthy nipple to create a new nipple after unilateral reconstruction. Even though this provides a perfect color match, the procedure can reduce or eliminate sensation and might affect the ability to breastfeed with the only fully functional nipple remaining after unilateral mastectomy. If you're considering nipple sharing, ask your surgeon how your healthy nipple will be affected.

Aftercare. You may not be impressed with your nipples when you first see them. They'll be red, swollen, and crisscrossed with dark stitches. Scabs form during the first couple of weeks. In about a month, soft, natural-looking nipples emerge from the scabby cocoon. It can be a shock when you first see them—they'll be almost twice as large as you might expect them to be. Supersizing them is deliberate: they shrink considerably as they heal and continue to flatten over several months. Soon they'll be much smaller and in better proportion to your breast. Try not to put any direct pressure on your delicate new nipples before they heal, because that might squash them. You can wear a lightweight bra while the nipple is healing, as long as it doesn't apply too much pressure. Don't shower or involve your nipples in sexual activity until your surgeon gives you the okay. Any mild discomfort (remember, there are no nerves in the new nipple) can be managed with over-the-counter analgesics. No matter which technique is used, your nipple needs a healthy blood supply to survive. Avoid smoking, caffeine, aspirin, and other blood-thinning medications for a few weeks before and after your nipple procedure.

*Wow! My new nipple is amazing! It matches my other nipple almost
exactly. The only way it could be better is if it had feeling.* —*Karla*

A Colorful Finish

In 8 to 12 weeks, the new nipple is fully healed and ready for cosmetic *tattooing*, the final step in the reconstructive process (figure 11.2). Even though tattooing doesn't create texture or projection, it adds a dramatic and real-

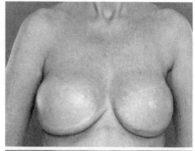

istic finish to your reconstructed breast by darkening the nipple and the skin around it to simulate an areola. If you're not ready at this point, or you're quite happy with the way your unpigmented nipples and areolae look, tattooing can be added anytime in the future. Or you can simply opt to forgo it altogether.

Who will create your tattoos? Tattooing is usually an in-office procedure performed by the surgeon or a member of his office staff. Some plastic surgeons contract with local tattoo artists, who often have a background in art and understand the subtle nuances of blending colors and shading for the most realistic effect. Research nipple tattooing as closely as you did your breast reconstruction, because if you're going to the trouble of having tattoos, you want them to be as good as possible. No matter who adds the pigment, ask about her

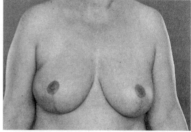

FIGURE 11.2. Before (*top*) and after (*bottom*) nipples are created and tattooed on reconstructed breast mounds. *Images provided by Dr. Frank J. DellaCroce and The Center for Restorative Breast Surgery, LLC.*

specific experience coloring reconstructed nipples and review before-and-after photos of her work. Speak with some of her previous reconstruction patients, if possible, to see whether they're happy with the results. If you're looking for something out of the ordinary, it may be worth your time to consult with a professional tattoo artist; many provide no-cost services for mastectomy patients (figure 11.3).

Choosing your colors. Whoever does your tattoos, discuss color selec-

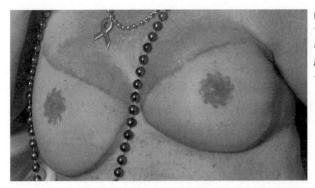

FIGURE 11.3. Some women prefer more artsy tattoos. *Image provided by Amy E. Burgess.*

tion before tattooing begins. You can choose from numerous shades of beige, brown, tan, pink, and rose. After unilateral mastectomy, you can match the color to your natural nipple. If you have bilateral reconstruction, some professionals recommend matching the natural color of your lips. Or bring a pre-op photo of your natural breasts as a reference. Blending two or more shades sometimes produces the most natural result. Combining rose with brown or adding beige and pink may give you the shade you want. Choose a hue that is somewhat darker than your final color—nipple tattoos fade as much as 40 to 50 percent. Review color samples with your tattoo professional and decide together which combination would best match your skin tone.

How it's done. Before your tattoo color is applied, your breast is swabbed with alcohol and the outline of your new areola is marked on the breast skin. Check the markings in a mirror before the tint is applied to be sure you approve of the position, shape, and size. If you had unilateral nipple reconstruction, the outlined area should match your natural areola. If both breasts are to be colored, the markings should be centered. If you don't like what you see, it's easy work to change the markings. If you're dissatisfied with the final tattoo, it's fairly simple to enlarge or recolor a tattoo—it's not as easy to make it smaller or lighter.

Once you've approved the initial outline, the tattooing can begin. The colors you selected are loaded into an electric tattoo gun, which holds sterilized needles. The color is delivered in a series of short bursts that inject the color under the skin within the previously marked area. The color is a bit shocking when you first see it: it looks like thick, shiny paint.

Because of reduced sensation in your breast, you'll probably feel more pressure or tingling than pain; you may feel a slight stinging. The longer you wait after your reconstruction, the more likely you'll feel the process, because you'll have regained some sensation. A local anesthesia isn't usually necessary; however, it can be applied if tattooing is too uncomfortable—and that's actually good news: it means you've kept or regained feeling in the front of your breast. Once under the skin, the color will fade to a more subtle shade. You may need to go back for another application of color to darken the area, create the desired shade, or fill in uneven spots.

Aftercare. It takes about 15 to 20 minutes to color each breast. Your newly tattooed nipples will initially appear darker and more red than they'll be when they're healed. (The red is from blood that mingles with the tattoo color.) Your new nipples and areolae will be covered with antibiotic ointment and a light bandage; you should receive aftercare instructions to take home with you. There's no downtime from tattooing, so you should be fine to return to work or home or go off to lunch or a meeting the same day. In four or five days, a scab will form over the tattooed area and then fall off. Take care not to rub, scrub, or pick at it, because that can create splotchy, uneven color.

Problems and Solutions

Although some nipple reconstructions fail, serious problems are rare when nipples are made of healthy skin. Complications that do occur usually involve cosmetic issues that are easily corrected. Infections and wound healing problems occur more frequently in irradiated skin.

Unsatisfactory pigmentation. Poorly distributed color can create a splotchy, uneven appearance that can be corrected by repeating the tattoo. Eventually, all body tattoos fade somewhat, but after three or four years, only the slightest hint of color may be all that remains of your nipple and areola. While this is a common problem, certain conditions accelerate fading. Nipple tattoos are typically a combination of red and brown, colors that diminish more noticeably than the blues, greens, and blacks used in many body tattoos. The type of pigment and tool used to implant the color can make a difference; having a local anesthetic can also inhibit color saturation. Your skin quality may also affect the longevity of your tattoo: radiation-treated skin or scar tissue often doesn't hold color well, for example. Chlorine can prematurely fade the color, so you'll need to avoid swimming pools and hot tubs for about six weeks after your color is applied. Sun exposure also accelerates fading.

> *When I first saw my new nipples, I thought my plastic surgeon had made a mistake. They seemed huge in proportion to my breasts. But they kept shrinking as they healed and after a few weeks they were the small nipples I had hoped for. When I later had them tattooed, I thought the tattoo artist had applied too much color. They were several shades darker than I had imagined. Once again, they faded as they healed. Unfortunately, they kept fading, and four years later, they're barely visible. The only thing I can do is have them re-tattooed but I just don't want to bother.*   —Kim

Poor position. The best way to avoid off-center nipples and areolae is to wait until your reconstructed breast is fully healed before having nipple surgery and to be sure you approve of the positional markings before the pigment is applied.

Nipple collapse. A reconstructed nipple may lose projection and flatten within a few weeks or few years of surgery. This is more likely when the skin at the donor site is thin. Radiation, scar tissue, and trauma can also cause a nipple to flatten. The solution is to recreate the nipple using a local flap or to plump it with synthetic tissue or cartilage. Many surgeons use an acellular dermal matrix when creating the nipple, to avoid this issue. Plastic surgeons at Memorial-Sloan Kettering Cancer Center have had good results by injecting Artecoll—a permanent soft tissue filler used to improve acne scars and fill wrinkles—into reconstructed nipples.[1] After three months of study on women who had nipple reconstruction with Artecoll, the material was entirely replaced by the body's own collagen. Nine months after the initial injections, all of the women in the study retained nipple projection.

Nipple failure. All or part of a reconstructed nipple may fail if the blood supply is inadequate. This happens more often with skin grafts than flaps. The resolution is to repeat the nipple reconstruction with a new flap.

Non-surgical Alternatives

If you decide not to have nipple reconstruction, you might want to use stick-on polyurethane or silicone semi-erect nipple prostheses, putting them on and taking them off whenever the mood strikes you. Rub-On Nipples (www.tattoonednipples.com) are another temporary way to have nipples when you want them and forgo them when you don't. If you have one healthy breast and one reconstructed breast, using these products will give you an even appearance. Several companies customize prosthetic nipples in different sizes and skin tones, including the little goosebumps on the areola known as Montgomery's tubercles; the companies include Reforma (www.myreforma.com), New Attitude (www.new-attitude-inc .com), Anaplastic Prosthetics (www.anaplastics.com), and Designed Medical Elements (https://nippleprosthetics.com).

Another option is having nipple and areola tattoos applied to your breast mounds. Simulating an areola with a tattoo and adding a smaller dark circle in the center creates the illusion of protrusion. It's not as realistic as a three-dimensional nipple, but it's an acceptable option for many women. Many tattoo professionals specialize in nipple and areola tattoos. They're experts in blending different shades to create a three-dimensional effect, so it looks as though you have nipples even when you don't.

PART THREE ○ PREP, POST-OP, RECOVERY, AND BEYOND

CHAPTER TWELVE

Preparing for Your Surgery

A woman is like a tea bag. You never know how strong she is until she gets into hot water. —ELEANOR ROOSEVELT

By now, you've done all your research and seen all the photos. You've talked to your surgeon about your reconstruction; you understand how it will be done and know what to expect. Your surgery date is circled in red on the kitchen calendar. There's a lot to be done before then, and now's the time to start.

Countdown: Four Weeks to Surgery

Your surgeon will provide a list of pre-op instructions, but generally, here's what you can expect within a month of your initial reconstruction surgery.

Finalize payment arrangement. Ideally, you should have written confirmation of your health insurer's payment authorization or have a payment plan in place with your plastic surgeon. If you've petitioned your insurance company for approval well in advance, this will, hopefully, not be an issue.

Take good care of yourself. Surgery is an assault on the body and its defenses, and fatigue is one of the most common side effects of general anesthesia. Up to this point, you've had to deal with many stressful decisions and issues; all this takes a toll on your mental and physical strength. If you've also undergone chemo or radiation—and perhaps both—your resiliency has been further weakened. Now more than ever, your body needs special care to prepare for surgery and improve your ability to recover. This is no time to try that new diet. Eat balanced meals with plenty of fruits, vegetables, and lean protein—meats, poultry, fish, and low-fat or nonfat dairy products are good sources. Drink plenty of fluids. Avoid alcohol or drink moderately. Try to sleep for eight hours each night.

Get in shape. Combined with balanced nutrition, increasing your fitness will help your body weather the stress of surgery. Exercise vigorously for at least 30 minutes a day (45 minutes to an hour is even better).

- Enjoy a brisk walk each morning or evening.
- Walk, swim, dance, try a new exercise DVD, or engage in other aerobic exercise to boost your immune system and strengthen your lungs and heart.
- Lift light weights to strengthen and tone the muscles of your shoulders and arms. You can also do push-ups, sit-ups, or other similar exercises, using your own body weight as resistance.
- Add sit-ups, abdominal crunches, and other exercises to strengthen your abdomen, if that will be a donor site.
- Give yoga a try. Yoga is a particularly effective way to improve the mind-body connection. Regularly stretching the muscles increases flexibility, resilience, and range of motion and is beneficial before and after surgery. Yoga also calms anxiety, increases blood flow, and can relieve postoperative discomfort. Done correctly, it strengthens lung capacity and respiratory function, which will help you recover from your surgery. Always start slowly and learn from a qualified instructor. Check with yoga studios, gyms, or the YWCA for nearby classes.

Breathe deeply. Our bodies breathe reflexively. We don't have to think about breathing for it to occur. Consciously inhaling and exhaling expands the lungs, bringing more oxygen into the body. Deep breathing clears the mind and offers new perspective. It's an effective way to restore calm after a stressful day or to counter pre-surgery jitters. Make a point of breathing deeply several times each day. You don't need any special equipment. Do it for five minutes before you get dressed, whenever you have a few minutes during the day, or just before you go to sleep. Lie on your back with one hand on your abdomen and the other on your chest. Slowly breathe in as much air as you can. Your lower hand will rise as your abdomen inflates with air. Breathe in slowly through your nose for four counts. Gradually exhale through your mouth for four counts, feeling your abdomen lower. Repeat four or five times.

Prepare emotionally. Many well-documented studies show that people who are emotionally prepared for surgery have less pain and heal sooner. Deal with stress and anxiety proactively. Try deep breathing exercises or meditation, or take a walk. Relaxation tapes and positive visualization are also helpful. *Prepare for Surgery, Heal Faster* by Peggy Huddleston (www .healfaster.com) is an excellent resource. If you've always thought about starting a journal, now is a great time. Sometimes it's easier to express your feelings to a non-judgmental piece of paper or a computer screen—it's also satisfying. You might be surprised at the depth of perspective it provides. Keep visual reminders of your post-reconstruction goals at hand. Hang photos of a smiling and happy you on the refrigerator as reminders that you'll be just fine after reconstruction. We all need something to look forward to, especially during trying times: stick a family picture or travel brochure for a post-reconstruction vacation or other future event to the mirror or prop it up on your desk.

> *Alone in my house, I cried all day. I was thankful for reconstruction, but I just couldn't come to grips with the reality of losing my breasts. My husband became so frustrated when he couldn't comfort me, he broke down and cried too. That was the day I decided I was done crying.* —Kathy

Stop smoking. You must be free of nicotine for at least three or four weeks before and after your surgery. That means no cigarettes, chewing tobacco, nicotine patches, or nicotine gum. You also need to stay away from secondhand smoke. This could be the push you need to quit for good. If you continue to smoke, your surgery may be delayed.

Two Weeks before Surgery

Understand the process and your instructions. Your surgeon will probably discuss the following issues (and more) with you before your operation. If he doesn't, be sure to ask him to do so.

- How long will my surgery last?
- How long will I stay in the hospital?
- Do I need to buy a special postoperative bra or camisole?
- What medications will I need at home and how long will I take them?
- How long until I may shower or bathe?
- What restrictions will I have during recovery?
- When will I be able to drive?
- When will my stitches be removed?
- When is my next office appointment after I'm discharged from the hospital?

Have pre-op testing. About two or three weeks before your operation, your surgeon will order routine preliminary tests to make sure you're healthy enough for surgery. Your pre-op tests may include:

- a blood test to check your red and white blood cell counts
- a chest x-ray
- an electrocardiogram to check your heart rhythm
- a stress echocardiogram to test your heart strength, if you had chemotherapy, have high blood pressure, have a family history of heart disease, or are age 55 or older
- an MRI or CT scan of your abdomen or buttocks, if they are donor sites
- additional tests, depending on your overall health, breast cancer diagnosis, and reconstructive procedure

Recruit help. Never underestimate the power and support of those who care about you. Recruit loved ones to care for your children, pets, and home during your recovery. When friends ask how they can help, suggest they babysit your kids, grocery shop, mow the lawn, run other errands, schedule a meal brigade, or drive you to doctor appointments. Let others help. Arrange for someone to drive you to the hospital and take you home. You'll also need someone to stay with you for at least the first 48 hours, and for several days if you have abdominal surgery.

Discontinue certain medications or supplements. Your surgeon will tell you which, if any, medications, vitamins, herbs, or supplements you should stop taking now and for a few weeks after your surgery. Taking aspirin, ibuprofen, or naproxen, which can thin the blood and inhibit clotting, is a definite no-no at least two weeks before and after surgery. You'll need to stay away from medications that include these ingredients, including many common non-prescription medications such as Advil, Aleve, Alka-Seltzer, Motrin, and others. When in doubt, read the label. Use Tylenol (acetaminophen) for relief from a headache, sore muscles, or other minor pain. If you're taking Coumadin (warfarin) or another blood thinner, your doctor may request a blood test just before your surgery to make sure your blood clots sufficiently. If you're taking tamoxifen or hormone replacement therapy, he might advise you to temporarily stop before and after your surgery, as both have the potential to promote bleeding and swelling.

Donate blood. Blood loss is minimized during reconstructive surgery and transfusions aren't usually required. If your surgery is a particularly long flap procedure or you have a history of bleeding problems, your surgeon will discuss the option to give blood beforehand. Then, in the unlikely event that you'll need it, your own blood will be used rather than donor blood.

Go shopping. You won't be able to bring a nightgown from home, but if you want to wear something more personal (and prettier) than a standard hospital gown, one option is to buy an Annie and Isabel designer hospital gown (www.annieandisabel.com). Designed by two nurses, the gowns have an inside pocket and snaps at the shoulders for easy access to surgery sites, and they conform to hospital standards. You may also need to shop for a post-op bra. Your surgeon will describe the type you should wear after your surgery. He may provide one for you in the hospital or request that you bring it with you. Bring this topic up if he doesn't mention it—you won't feel like wandering through the mall once you're released from the hospital. This is also a good time to shop for comfy camisoles, loose clothing that fastens in the front, or pretty new pajamas (silk or satin fabrics will make it easier to slide in and out of bed). You may also want to order a special belt to hold surgical drains (as described in chapter 14). Some women suggest buying underwear a size or two larger than you normally wear to accommodate swelling if you're having an abdominal or gluteal flap, although your surgeon will provide a compression girdle that you'll need to wear for several weeks.

Fill prescriptions. Your surgeon will prescribe pain medication and antibiotics for you to take once you return home. It's a good idea to have those prescriptions filled now, before you go to the hospital. If you think you'll have trouble getting to sleep the night before your surgery, request a mild sleeping medication. This is also a good time to refill any other medications you routinely take, so you'll have an ample supply during your recovery. After mastectomy, it will be painful to press down sufficiently to open childproof lids, so ask your pharmacist to use a different type of lid on your prescription bottles.

One Week to Go

Provide pre-admitting information. You'll have a mountain of paperwork to fill out before you enter the operating room. Your hospital may ask you to fill out several forms before your scheduled surgery date, or someone from the hospital's administrative staff may contact you to obtain all the necessary data ahead of time.

Pamper yourself. Now is a great time to get your hair cut and colored, have a facial, or engage in your favorite self-indulgent behavior. Have lunch with friends. Finish that big project at home or work. Go shopping. Take your kids on a trip. Have fun. Consider having your underarms and legs waxed—you may not be able to shave for two or three weeks after surgery.

Notify your surgeon of any health problems. Between now and your surgery date, notify your surgeon's office if you get a cold, infection, fever, cold sores, or other health problem, no matter how minor it may seem. Your surgery may have to be rescheduled if there is risk of infection—it's always better to be safe than sorry.

If you're a mom, discuss your impending absence and recovery with your kids. Many women feel it is better to tell their children about reconstruction instead of keeping it a secret. Children know when something is wrong, even if they don't know what it is, and they want to be reassured that their world will remain unchanged. Kids process information differently. Some ask lots of questions, while others aren't interested, so it's a good idea to tailor your explanations to each child's personality and level of understanding. Your demeanor influences their reaction: if they see you're okay, they'll be okay. Keep it simple for little ones, and give them only the details they need to understand why you'll be gone for a few days. If they don't already know about your breast cancer and treatment, reassure them you're not ill because of anything they did. Some women prefer to avoid using the word "sick," which may frighten children.

Keep your children's routines as normal as possible. Explain to little ones that you won't be able to pick them up for a while and that they must be careful not to jump on you when you come home. If you're emotional around your children, explain that you feel sad or angry or afraid, but not because of them. Older children and teens will want to know more. They may feel frightened or threatened if they sense reconstruction is a taboo topic. Reassure them that you'll be fine and that your reconstruction is a way to help restore your breast after mastectomy. Let them know how they can help during your recovery.

My four-year-old had already seen me bald and sick after chemotherapy, so when I told him I was going back to the hospital for a few days to get better, he didn't even blink. —Christine

Our puppy had to have surgery after he swallowed pillow stuffing. When I scheduled my mastectomy, I explained that Mommy's boobs had a type of stuffing that could make me sick, so a nice doctor was going to replace the bad stuffing with good stuffing. I would be in the hospital, as our puppy had, and then I would come home and soon be all better. I gave each of my children a teddy bear I said was filled with "Mommy love" that would never run out. Whenever I couldn't hug them, they could cuddle the bears and it would be like me giving them a big squeeze. —Cathy

Catch up, stock up. A little preparation now will make things easier on you and your family when you come home from the hospital.

- Shop for groceries and stock up on fresh fruits and vegetables, juices, and items that are easy for someone else to prepare. Stash a batch of reheatable meals in the freezer. This is especially important if you don't have someone who can deliver meals or shop and cook for you during your recovery. Have small bags of ice or frozen food on hand to wrap in a towel and apply to reduce swelling. Don't forget supplies for your pets.
- Buy a thermometer if you don't already have one. It will come in handy if you think you might have a fever.
- Check your camera batteries if you'd like to keep a photo journal of your recovery, as many women do.
- Clean your house or have it cleaned before you go into the hospital. You won't be able to sweep or push a vacuum for several weeks.
- Catch up on the laundry.

Prepare for recovery. Do as much as possible now to prepare for your recovery.

- List chores and errands that other family members will need to take care of, such as paying bills, shopping for groceries, taking the kids to and from school and sports activities, and changing the litter box.
- Make a contact list of telephone numbers or e-mail addresses of friends and family who should be notified after your surgery and kept posted on your recovery.
- Arrange your nightstand with all the things you'll need once you get home, including pain medication, TV and DVD remote controls, books and magazines, tissues, lotion, and telephone (if you want it). Baby wipes are handy for the times when you just won't feel like getting up— although periodically getting up and walking around is good for you. You'll also want to have water and saltines or graham crackers handy for taking pain medication in the middle of the night. Keep a digital tablet, journal and pen, or small tape recorder handy if you're inclined to document your thoughts.
- Reposition bathroom and kitchen counter items so you can get to them easily without reaching—lifting your arms or stretching them up over your head is something you won't be doing for a while after you get home. If you're having an abdominal flap, do the same with items

positioned under cabinets and on low shelves, so you can get to them without bending.

- Ask friends not to call for a few days after you come home from the hospital. Having the phone ring just when you drop off to sleep can be very disrupting. If you feel like talking, you can always call them. You can also turn down or turn off the ringer or simply unplug the phone so you won't be disturbed.

The Day before Surgery

Remove any nail polish and artificial nails. The nail of your index or middle finger on each hand should be *au naturel* when you go into surgery. (Your preoperative instructions may request that you remove all nail polish.) Your anesthesiologist will clip a monitor onto the end of a finger to determine whether you're getting enough oxygen while you're asleep.

Relax in your favorite way. See a movie with friends, have dinner with your family or your favorite person, get a massage, or put on some music and stretch out in a warm bath. Engage in your favorite stress-reducing activity.

Wash with antibacterial soap. Cleanse your entire chest, sides, underarms, and donor site with Hibiclens or Dial over-the-counter antibacterial soap to eliminate bacteria on your skin and reduce the likelihood of infection.

Decide what you'll wear to and from the hospital. Select something that is comfortable, is easy to get on and off, and doesn't need to be pulled over your head. Wear sweatpants, pajama bottoms, or other loose comfy pants, especially if you're having abdominal or gluteal surgery. Wear slippers or flat-heeled shoes.

Pack a small overnight bag. Take moisturizer, lip gloss or balm, toothbrush, floss, hairbrush or comb, and any other essentials. The hospital will supply a toothbrush and toothpaste (for a charge), but you can bring your own if you prefer. The hospital will also provide slippers and a robe, but you can bring your own instead. It's also nice to pack your favorite music, e-reader, or books-on-tape, particularly if you'll be in the hospital for several days. Don't forget a sports bra if your surgeon recommended one. And remember your insurance card, personal identification, and any paperwork your surgeon asked you to bring to the hospital, including copies of all your pre-op test results, even if copies were previously sent to him. Some patients appreciate having their own quilt in the hospital room, to make it seem a little bit more personal. Pack a special bag for your husband, partner, or family member, or whoever will accompany you to the hospital. They'll be spending long hours in the waiting room during your surgery. Include water, snacks, something to read, and a list of family and friends to notify after your surgery. Be sure to charge the cell phone or pack plenty of change for the pay phone.

Don't bring medications. There's no need to bring prescribed medications to the hospital. Your surgeon will order all the medicine you'll need during your hospital stay, including any prescribed by other doctors.

Talk to your anesthesiologist. If he hasn't already done so, your anesthesiologist may call to ask questions about your general health, allergies, and any past reactions you may have had to anesthesia. (Alternatively, he may see you in the hospital just before your surgery.) If you were nauseous after a prior general anesthetic, for example, he may include an extra dose of anti-nausea medication with your anesthesia.

Stay hydrated. Drink plenty of water and clear liquids throughout the day. Don't drink alcohol; it dries the tissues, and you need to be as hydrated as possible for your surgery. It may also interact with anesthesia or postoperative painkillers.

Eat a light dinner. Enjoy a light, low-fiber dinner tonight to discourage post-op intestinal gas and nausea. Don't eat or drink anything, including gum, candy, or water, after midnight or the cutoff time advised by your anesthesiologist. Patients should always go into surgery with an empty stomach, to avoid the possibility of vomiting. If your surgery is scheduled for the afternoon, your anesthesiologist may approve Gatorade, water, apple juice, or other clear beverage. Always follow her instructions.

Make love, if you feel like it. If you're so inclined, there's no medical reason to avoid sex the night before your surgery. It may even help calm your nerves.

Try for eight hours of sleep. With your surgery looming, you'll have a lot on your mind. Try to get a good night's rest. If you think that's not going to be possible on your own, ask your doctor to prescribe a mild sedative. Don't take an over-the-counter sleep aid unless you have his okay.

Plant positive thoughts. Before you drift off to sleep, tell yourself that your surgery will be successful, you'll come through it beautifully, and you'll be just fine. Then believe it.

It's Reconstruction Day

Take your regular medication. By now, you should have spoken to your surgeon about the medications you take. If he approved you to do so, take your regular medication with just enough water to swallow.

Shower, wash, and shave. Thoroughly wash all surgical areas again with antibacterial soap. This is the last chance to wash your hair for several days. Use an electric razor to shave your underarm or legs, or be very careful if you use a safety razor—any nick or cut may invite infection.

Leave it all off. Don't apply wigs, hairpieces, creams, lotions, perfume, or makeup (your natural skin tone is an indication of adequate circulation). Bring your eyeglasses if you need them; you cannot wear contact lenses during surgery and you won't feel like putting them in and taking them out during recovery in the hospital.

Leave all valuables at home. Don't take anything you don't need. Leave cash, credit cards, your purse, wallet, watch, and all jewelry, including wedding rings, earrings, and body jewelry, at home.

Talk to someone. Chat with your kids, your spouse, your significant other, or your best friend. It will help to quiet any concerns they're having. It will help you too.

Leave little notes. If you have kids, tuck a note from Mom under their pillow or somewhere they'll be sure to find it, so they'll have a message from you even when you're not there.

Try to relax. It's natural to be nervous before surgery. But you can take steps to calm your thoughts and fears. Plant positive thoughts about your surgery, recovery, and outcome. Lie flat on the floor, close your eyes, breathe deeply, and focus on the most positive, beautiful thoughts you can—a happy time, a romantic vacation, or giggling with your children. Visualize a peaceful, happy postoperative you.

CHAPTER THIRTEEN

What to Expect in the Hospital

A good laugh and a long sleep are the best cures in the doctor's book. —IRISH PROVERB

Who doesn't get the jitters just walking into a hospital? It's a place we associate with the sick and ailing. Knowing what to expect once you're within those sanitized walls can help calm your fear of the unknown.

Admitting and Pre-op

The hospital will want you to arrive two to three hours before your surgery. Once there, you'll be asked to review and sign a pile of paperwork, including the following:

- A general information form that lists your name, address, health insurance information, surgeon, primary care doctor, and next of kin.
- A questionnaire about your medical history. You'll be asked to provide information about your allergies, previous surgeries, whether you smoke or not, and other similar information. By this time, you may have provided this same information several times for various doctors; however, this is an important precaution. The hospital doesn't want to give you Demerol for your pain if it makes you sick or penicillin for an infection if you're allergic to it.
- Notification that you've received a copy of the Patient's Bill of Rights, a document that outlines the hospital's responsibilities and your rights.
- A surgical consent form identifying the procedure to be performed and the name of your surgeon. Be sure you read this and verify the information. Signing the form also means you understand the potential risks of the operation.
- A power of attorney form, identifying your designated appointee to

make financial and other decisions on your behalf, if necessary. This can be unnerving, but don't fear. It's a formality, just in the very unlikely event something untoward happens to you during surgery.

- Authorization for the hospital to provide you with blood from its supply, if necessary, unless you've donated your own blood before surgery. This is rarely needed for mastectomy or reconstructive operations.

A nurse will show you to your room, and you'll change into a hospital gown. She'll weigh you, take your blood pressure, and ask you to remove hearing aids, dentures, prosthetic limbs, contact lenses, or any other artificial apparatus.

Each time I entered the hospital for a blood test, my hands began to shake and a feeling of dread came over me. I had to find a more positive perspective to get through my reconstruction. I began to consider hospitals and doctors as places and people who did things for me rather than to me. I started to consider reconstruction as the process that would put me back on the road to wholeness.   *—Dorene*

While you're waiting, your general surgeon and plastic surgeon will come by to chat with you before you enter the OR. If your plastic surgeon hasn't already marked the incision reference lines on your chest and donor site, she'll draw them now. The anesthesiologist will stop by to introduce himself and review your medical history. Once you're on the operating table, he'll mix up a custom anesthesia just for you, based on your weight and the length of your surgery.

There's always a lot of waiting around before surgery. Free to wander, your mind may go directly to uneasy. Breathe deeply. Concentrate on the positive aspects of your surgery. Mastectomy will remove your cancer (or most of the threat of cancer) and reconstruction will restore your breasts. Don't keep your fears to yourself. If it will make you feel better, discuss them with your doctors, your husband or partner, family members, or others who are in the hospital with you or are just a telephone call away.

I was so nervous the day of my surgery, I broke into a cold sweat. I remember wondering if I would be admitted for heart problems instead

of reconstruction, because I was sure I could feel my heart hammering
beneath my shirt.   —*Jasmine*

Showtime in the OR

When it's time for your surgery, friends and family will be shown to the
waiting room, and you'll be taken to the operating room on a gurney (a
bed with wheels). In some private or small facilities, you may simply walk
in. The first thing you'll notice is the temperature, which is deliberately kept
low for the surgical staff. Their tightly woven gowns that protect against
bacteria are made with a fabric that doesn't breathe, and the room lights
generate plenty of heat. A nurse will cover you immediately with heated
blankets, and pre-surgery preparations begin. Small sensors will be taped
to your arms and legs to monitor your pulse, blood pressure, heart rate, and
the level of oxygen in your blood.

It's natural to feel anxious at this point, but it won't last long—you'll soon
be fast asleep. You'll feel a small sting (similar to having your blood drawn)
as the anesthesiologist inserts a thin needle into a vein on the inside of
your arm or on the top of your hand. Through this intravenous (IV) tube,
he'll administer a complex and precise anesthesia directly into your bloodstream. He may give you a sedative first. You'll be asleep before you can
count to 10 . . . and maybe before you get to 5.

The technology of modern anesthesia is really quite sophisticated. Yet
when patients are asked what they fear most about surgery, many say it's
the anesthesia. They're afraid they'll overdose or wake up during the operation in horrible pain. In fact, the anesthesiologist closely adjusts the mix-
ture you receive at all times during your surgery, to prevent either of these
mishaps. He monitors your vital signs and carefully controls your level of
consciousness, administering a precise dose of sedative to keep you in a
deep sleep. Not too much, not too little—just enough. Many patients fear
they'll talk in their sleep, divulging some deep, dark secret once they're
under, but that's not likely.

Once asleep, you'll receive pain medication, so you won't feel a thing
during surgery. A surgical tube will be placed in your throat to help you
breathe and a urinary catheter will be inserted into your bladder to drain

your urine. A nurse will wash your chest and donor site with surgical disinfectant. The rest of your body will be draped with sterile sheets, leaving only the surgical areas uncovered. The general surgeon begins your mastectomy as described in chapter 4. The plastic surgeon then moves in to do the reconstruction.

A Peek into Post-op

When your surgery is over, you'll be wheeled into the recovery room, and your surgeon will let your loved ones know your operation has been completed.

In recovery. As the effects of anesthesia begin to wear off, you'll slowly wake up, but you'll be drowsy and will continue to fall in and out of sleep. You'll have surgical drains at your incision sites (more about these in chapter 14), and you may have an oxygen tube in your nose when you awake. When you're breathing well enough to inhale sufficient oxygen into your system, the *pulse oximeter* clamp on your finger—put there to monitor the level of oxygen in your blood—will be removed. An IV will drip saline and antibiotics into your bloodstream. Your nurse will give you ice chips if your mouth is dry and warm blankets if you're chilled. Pressurized elastic stockings on your legs will help prevent blood clots until you're able to move around—you'll feel a gentle pressure and hear a soft whooshing sound as the pumping machine periodically compresses the stockings to mimic normal circulation. Your breasts will be encased in a surgical bra or compression garment like an elastic tube top, and your donor site will be bandaged. You may be curious and perhaps anxious to see what's under your bandage; unless you get an upside-down peek while a nurse is checking your incisions, you won't see what's under the dressing until it's removed in your doctor's office in a few days.

Initially, the pain medication administered during surgery should take care of your post-op pain. The nurse can give you additional pain medication if you need it and anti-nausea medicine if your stomach is upset. After implant or expander reconstruction, you'll soon be moved to your hospital room, usually for an overnight stay. (Some women go home the same day; others remain in the hospital for a second night, depending on how their recovery goes.) If you've had flap surgery, a Doppler probe will be implanted into your new breast so that nurses can closely monitor blood flow to the flap during your first few days in the hospital.

In your room. Anesthesia suppresses the body's ability to function normally. You'll feel weak and tired and your head may feel fuzzy for the next 24 to 48 hours, until its effects wear off. The longer you're under the influence of the anesthesia, the harder your body needs to work to recover. You'll be very thirsty from the anesthesia, and your throat may be sore from the breathing tube. Ask your nurse for water, juice, or throat lozenges. She'll frequently check your temperature, blood pressure, pulse, and heart rate and will empty your surgical drains. To be sure you remain comfortable, she'll also regularly ask you to assess your level of pain. You'll have a call button or an intercom to summon your nurse whenever you need help.

Your bed will be angled to elevate your chest, so you'll be reclining in a semi-upright position. If you had reconstruction with an abdominal flap, the lower portion of the bed will be positioned to lessen tension on your donor incision. The urinary catheter will still be in your bladder, so you won't immediately have to get up to urinate. By judging the amount of urine you produce, your nurse can ensure you're not dehydrated. Some women don't even feel the catheter. Others say it makes them feel they have to urinate when they don't. It stays in place until you can walk to the bathroom on your own. Constipation is a common problem after general anesthesia; you may not have a bowel movement for three to five days following surgery. Eating lightly the day before your surgery will help to avoid a bloated feeling. Walking, drinking plenty of clear fluids, and eating sufficient fiber will help get you back on track. Ask the nurse for a stool softener if you need it.

Your First Day after Surgery

A ventilating machine breathed for you while you were in surgery, and now it's important to get your lungs back up to full capacity. You'll be given a *spirometer* to help expand your lungs and strengthen your breathing. It's a plastic box divided into three separate chambers, each with a small ball.

To use it, you first exhale to expel the air in your lungs. Then, as you inhale through the mouthpiece, your lungs expand. Each ball rises independently and stays up as long as you hold your breath. At first, it will be difficult to elevate even the first ball. Practice hourly until you can keep all three balls at the top simultaneously. Don't skip this little exercise. Restoring lung strength is a very important part of your recovery.

Managing pain. Most women are concerned about the pain they'll experience after such major surgery, but many describe having more of a dull, heavy feeling than a sharp or unbearable pain. Of course, a lot depends on the type of reconstruction you've had and how well you recover. To better understand the source of your pain, consider this: You know how annoying a paper cut can be, and that affects only the top layer of skin. Your surgical incision is a paper cut magnified, slicing through skin, tissue, and muscle.

Contemporary medicine capably handles post-op pain no matter what type of reconstruction you have. Oral medication is usually adequate after implant or expander surgery. Flap surgery is more invasive and requires more substantial pain control, so when you awake from that surgery, you'll have a self-medicating pump that regulates the amount of medication you receive—you can use it when you need it, without fear of overdosing. When the level of the pain significantly subsides, you'll be switched to oral pain-killers. Many surgeons now also place an On-Q Painbuster during flap surgery. It's a small, round pump that delivers local anesthetic through a thin tube directly to your surgical site (see an animation of how this works at www.iflo.com). If this adequately controls your discomfort, you won't be as groggy, drowsy, or constipated as you would be with the stronger narcotic dispensed by other pain management methods. The trick to managing pain is to stay ahead of it by keeping a constant, even flow of medication in your system. Allow 15 to 20 minutes for the medication to kick in; dose yourself *before* the pain is excruciating. This is no time to be tough—patients who control their pain heal faster than those who don't. At this point, your fresh incisions are tender and sensitive, and applying pressure to them, either internally or externally, will hurt. A sneeze or cough will feel like a grenade going off inside. Holding your hand or a pillow gently against your incisions will help. Try to support your incisions in the same way when you get in or out of bed.

Circulation and movement. Movement improves circulation, prevents fluid from settling in your lungs, and helps your system return to normal. As you rest in bed, periodically rotate your ankles and gently stretch your arms and legs. Slowly and carefully flex and stretch as many body parts as you can without causing pain. Don't use your arms, chest, or shoulders until your surgeon says it's okay—you'll initially have limited mobility in your arms, and if lymph nodes were removed during your mastectomy, your underarms may be tender.

Getting out of bed for the first time will be an effort, particularly if you have an abdominal incision, but the sooner you're mobile, the sooner you'll be on the way to recovery. It's very important to walk around and get your blood circulating, even if just for a few moments. The sooner you can become somewhat mobile, the sooner you can go home. With most types of reconstruction, you'll be encouraged to get out of bed the day after your surgery; after implant or expander surgery, you may be up and walking the same day. Start by sitting up carefully with the help of the nurse. Take a few steps around the room or walk to the bathroom. It will be difficult and exhausting the first time or two you try to get up. Try to get out of bed every few hours and take a short stroll or sit up in a chair. Each time will be easier as you regain strength. It's also easier to move around when you're not in pain, so for the first few days, be sure you're amply medicated before you get in and out of bed.

The Rest of Your Hospital Stay

Although your health insurance may dictate the length of your stay, all bodily functions must operate normally before you can leave the hospital. Talk with your doctor about staying longer if you don't feel well enough to go home or if you develop an infection.

When it's time to go home, be sure you leave the hospital with the following:

- instructions that explain how to care for your incisions
- a list of warning signs for infection or other problems
- directions for managing your surgical drains
- prescriptions for pain medication and antibiotics (if you don't already have them)
- out-of-hours contact information for your plastic surgeon
- a scheduled follow-up appointment with your surgeon

When you've packed up everything you need and your surgeon has signed your discharge papers, a nurse will help you into a wheelchair and take you outside. (For insurance reasons, patients aren't allowed to walk out of the hospital.) You're on your way home.

CHAPTER FOURTEEN

Back Home

Today is the first day of the rest of your life.

—ABBIE HOFFMAN

After surgery, your definition of a good day will change as you recover and regain strength. At first, a good day will simply mean finding a comfortable sleeping position. That will be redefined when you can stay awake, sit up, respond to e-mails or texts, and have dinner with your family. Later, a good day will be one when you can lift your arms over your head or go the entire day without a nap. One day your cancer, treatment, reconstruction, and doctors' appointments will be behind you. You'll go about your life and forget about your chest, just as you did before your surgery. That will be a good day.

A Timetable for Healing

Just three months after losing his legs in an accident on the track, world champion race car driver Alex Zanardi was up and walking on artificial limbs. Zanardi said of his recovery, "The good thing is that I've turned the first page of that book. Actually, I've finished the first chapter. All of the others are very, very short." Now that's a positive outlook on recovery. If you can view your own reconstruction with the same outlook—the worst is behind you—it will be easier to keep the end result in view.

Once you return home, sleeping or resting will initially take up a large portion of your days. Though you'll be eager to return to your normal routine, don't rush your recovery. Give in to your need to rest. For the first few days, you won't be opening the refrigerator, cutting a loaf of bread, or making any movements that use your chest muscles—and that includes many of the things you're used to doing throughout the day. You'll feel very tired. Take advantage of the time to write in your journal, catch up on your reading, watch favorite movies, or just nap whenever you feel the need. Listen to your body and be respectful of your need to heal. As your body recuperates, so will your energy and spirit. Don't be frustrated when you can't reach the top shelf or blow-dry your hair. Day by day, you'll get better, and your functionality, strength, and range of motion will improve.

How long will it take to get back to normal? Recovery is such a personal matter, and it's different for everyone. A lot depends on your condition before surgery, the type of reconstruction you have—you'll bounce back faster after implant reconstruction than after a tissue flap—and how much you do to support the healing process. Here's a general description of what you can expect during the first few weeks. Your own recovery may move along faster or take a while longer.

Week 1. It's important to protect your chest in the days following your surgery. You'll need to move slowly and carefully—no extensive reaching, stretching, pulling, or pressing movements, nothing that puts too much stress on your tender chest tissue. You'll find out very quickly what you can and can't do (table 14.1). Try not to raise your arms above your head or behind your back—that's why front-closing pajamas or tops come in handy. You'll feel very tired and perhaps lightheaded during your first postoperative week. Even though you may spend much of the day in bed, you can dress (or stay in your comfy pajamas or nightgown), take short walks down the hall or around the house, sit up and watch TV, and take meals with the rest of the family. You'll be advised not to pick up anything weighing over five pounds—this includes children. If you've had an abdominal flap, your incision will keep you from standing up straight; you'll be hunched over when you walk, until you begin to heal.

Your hospital nurse should have given you instructions for taking care of your mastectomy dressing at home. It's important to keep it dry; a damp dressing encourages infection. Your surgeon may tell you it's fine to shower once you get home (some women, especially those whose incisions were closed with surgical glue, get the okay to shower while they're still in the hospital), as long as you don't let the water pound your incision. You may feel too tired to shower; some women find it helpful to sit on a shower stool. You may also want to ask someone to help you. If you decide to try a shower, turn your back to the water spray, or if you have an adjustable

TABLE 14.1. Recovery dos and don'ts

10 things you won't be able to do for a while	10 things you'll be able to do
1. Lift more than 5 pounds	1. Take naps
2. Scratch your back	2. Walk more each day
3. Reach over your head	3. Enjoy TV and movies
4. Sleep on your stomach	4. Send e-mails or texts
5. Exercise aerobically	5. Do range-of-motion exercises (when approved by doctor)
6. Vacuum or sweep	6. Knit or crochet
7. Take out the garbage	7. Have meals at home with family or friends
8. Open childproof or screw-top lids	8. Catch up on your reading
9. Style and/or color your hair	9. Use social media to update your status
10. Drive	10. Write thank-you cards to thoughtful friends

shower head, turn it to the gentlest setting. Be very careful, because you'll still be weak and your incision won't be completely healed. If the surgeon advises you to keep your incisions dry for a while longer, take sponge baths instead, or sit in a half-filled tub. Lightly pat your incisions dry, and leave the steri-strips (small tape) or surgical glue in place until they fall off on their own or your surgeon removes them. Wash with a soap that isn't harsh or scented. Avoid application of any lotions, creams, or powders to your incision, except antibacterial creams that your physician recommends.

It probably won't be your priority for several days, but when you can't wait to have clean hair—it's such a luxury—lean your neck carefully over the sink (if you can do it without pain) and have someone do the honors for you. Your clean hair may need to wait a while longer if you have an abdominal incision and can't manage this.

You'll have a post-op appointment with your plastic surgeon within a week of your surgery, to check your incisions and change your dressing. (You'll need someone to drive you there and back home.) This is a good time to ask for a copy of your post-mastectomy pathology report and make sure a copy was sent to your oncologist (if your mastectomy was treatment for breast cancer).

Know when to call your doctor. It's normal to have discomfort, soreness, and fatigue after surgery. Notify your doctor, however, if you experience any of the following symptoms:

- chills or a fever higher than 101 degrees
- persistent vomiting or nausea
- pale, blue, or cold fingers, toes, or nails
- increased numbness, tingling, or swelling in your fingers
- redness, warmth, or excessive firmness around your incision
- bleeding into your bandage that doesn't stop when pressure is applied to the incision for 10 minutes
- a cloudy discharge or foul odor at the incision site
- pain that isn't controlled by your prescribed medication

I always thought napping during the day was such a waste of time. After my surgery, I just gave in to it. I kept a pile of books by the bed. I would wake up, read a little, walk a little, then readjust my pillows and nod off again. How decadent! —Mona

Week 2. Most women find they can do more in the second week. After implant surgery, you may be feeling more like your old self by now, and although you may tire easily, you'll probably be able to stay awake longer during the day. If you've had reconstruction with an abdominal flap, make a concerted effort to stand a little bit straighter each day. Everything just takes longer and uses more energy.

This is the time when many women make the mistake of doing too much too soon. You won't feel like dancing yet, although you should feel better than you did in the first week. Move slowly and carefully and give yourself time to gradually get back into the swing of things. You're still recovering—never force your body to do something before it's ready. Add a few more minutes to your daily strolls, until you're walking for 10 to 15 minutes (or longer, if you can manage it) each time.

I was tired and fuzzy for a few days after my implant reconstruction; I was okay as long as I took my pain pills. I was so much better by the second week, I decided to shop for groceries. What a mistake! I was utterly exhausted in 10 minutes. I couldn't push the cart one more step. I left it right in the middle of the cereal aisle, got back into my car, and had a good cry. —Shelly

Week 3. By now you should be taking longer walks and staying up most of the day. You may still need a nap or two during the day to feel more alert and less fatigued. Until your incisions heal and your drains are removed, avoid activities that can raise your blood pressure, including sexual activity—excess blood at the incision can cause swelling and hinder healing. Depending on the type of reconstruction you had and how your recovery is progressing, your surgeon may give you the okay to start specific exercises. If you're well enough and off pain medication, he may also say it's okay to begin driving again, although it may be a bit longer until you're up to that. Do a test first: sit in a parked car and see whether you're able to open the car door without straining your chest muscles: get in and out, and turn the wheel. If it's too uncomfortable, wait another week or two. You'll need to cushion your breasts from the seat belt, whether you're a driver or a passenger. Placing a small pillow or a folded towel between the belt and your chest will do the trick.

If you've had a flap reconstruction, particularly an abdominal flap, you might feel you've hit a recovery plateau about this time. The fatigue, discomfort, trouble sleeping, and just being tired of recovering will catch up with you, and you'll feel weary of it all. You may be able to stand straight (or almost straight) by this time, even though your abdomen will continue to feel tight for a while longer. Realize it's temporary. Continue to take your naps and your walks, do the stretching exercises your doctor recommends, and tomorrow or the next day (or the day after that), you'll notice an improvement.

For the first couple weeks after my reconstruction I was constantly aware of the tightness in my chest, the feeling that something was different. Then at three weeks, I felt normal, just like I used to before surgery. It was a big deal; I was getting used to the new me. I felt so good, I made plans to go

*out on my own, but after just a few hours, I was so tired! I must have over-
done it because I needed a nap when I got home; most days I just needed to
sit down and relax for a while and then I would feel better. I also realized
that it was too soon for me to have been driving on my own. Resting after
going out seemed to be the routine until almost five weeks to the day, when
I started feeling that most of my energy had returned. My mom reminded
me that although I may have felt well during those early weeks, my body
was working very hard in the background . . . healing.*   —Lianne

Week 4. You'll probably be able to resume much of your normal routine
by this time (if you haven't already), particularly after implant or expander
surgery. If you've had a flap procedure—especially an attached TRAM—
or you've suffered healing problems, you may need extra time to recover.
It may be two to four more weeks before you're able to get back to most
normal activities, and it can be a few months before the tightness in your
abdomen disappears. If you stopped smoking, don't resume until this week
or until your doctor gives you permission. (You've now been off cigarettes
for six to eight weeks—a great start to kick the habit!) If you had flap reconstruction and your new breast isn't sore, your surgeon may say it's okay to
begin wearing ordinary bras.

Phantom sensations. As your nerves grow back, you may feel temporary tingling, shooting pains, or tickling, like the sensations when your foot
goes to sleep. Some women also experience phantom pains: itching or tingling where the breast used to be. People who lose limbs often report the
same phenomenon—it's your brain continuing to process routine signals
connected with sensations in the breast. In time, it will adjust to the fact
that the breast and nerves are no longer there, and the odd feelings will
subside and disappear. In the meantime, if your reconstructed breast itches,
scratching won't help, because you won't feel it. Try rubbing or scratching
nearby, where you do have feeling.

*After my mastectomy with DIEP reconstruction, I stayed in the hospital
for six days. Pain was minimal; I was off all pain meds, including ibuprofen, within a week. I ate meals with my family from my first day home*

and slept in my own bed—that was difficult since I had to sleep flat on my back for the first three weeks. Though I worried about how my kids (ages 15 months, 3, and 5) would handle my recovery, it went better than I expected. My healing was aided significantly by all the help I accepted, including meals, preschool rides, and a cleaning service. I was able to care for myself within 10 days of surgery, and I was completely back to normal within a month. The lifting restriction was the hardest part of the recovery process for me. As a stay-at-home mom, I wasn't able to lift my youngest in and out of the crib.　　　　　　　　　　　　　*—Jenni*

Cooking is my passion. During my recovery, I amassed a huge pile of new recipes from the TV cooking shows I watched all day. I couldn't wait to try them. I didn't consider myself to be back to normal until the fourth week after my operation when I could get back into the kitchen.　　　*—Verna*

Managing Medication

Your doctor will prescribe pain medication and antibiotics after your surgery. Take antibiotics at regular intervals throughout the day until you've finished all of them. If they make you nauseous, don't take Maalox, Mylanta, Tums, or other antacids, which may negate the effectiveness of the antibiotics. Ask your surgeon for a different prescription instead. Manage your medication with the following tips.

- Take your pain medication when you need it. Studies show that patients who manage their pain heal faster than those who don't. It's more effective to keep a level amount of pain medication in your system than to wait until your pain becomes unmanageable.
- Taper off. Take pain medication less frequently or take one pill instead of two (or a half instead of a whole pill) when you begin to feel better. When you think you can tolerate something less, switch to extra-strength Tylenol or whatever your doctor recommends.
- Prevent nausea. Take pain pills with milk or food to prevent nausea. Most antibiotics can be taken on an empty stomach or with food.
- Be prepared for a mid-evening dose of pain medication. In the first week

or two after surgery, your pain may wake you up during the night. Time your medication so you have one dose just before you go to bed. Keep water and saltines or graham crackers by your bed so you won't have to get up to take your medicine.

- Combat constipation. Pain medications and decreased mobility may leave you irregular, and straining from constipation puts added stress on abdominal incisions. Treating constipation preemptively will help to avoid the problem. Increase your daily fiber intake and stay hydrated. Iron promotes constipation—if you take a multivitamin, use one without iron until your bowels are back to normal. Frequent walking will also help restore your regularity. If your bowels refuse to cooperate, try Colace, Senekot, or other stool softener recommended by your doctor.
- Don't drive until you're no longer taking pain medication.
- Avoid alcohol. It exacerbates drowsiness from pain medication and can sometimes interfere with antibiotics.

Dealing with Drains

Surgical drains are grenade-shaped plastic bulbs with long tubing that is sutured under the skin at the incision sites (figure 14.1). Many women consider these to be the most annoying aspect of recovery. You'll be eager to get rid of these pesky contraptions; however, they aid healing by siphoning off fluids at the surgery sites. Just think what the post-surgical experience was like before someone invented these drains: all that fluid you empty out

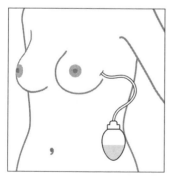

would otherwise accumulate in your body, promoting swelling and infection and delaying healing. Until the early 1990s, patients stayed in the hospital until their drains were removed. Today, shorter hospital stays are emphasized and drains are easily managed at home.

Drains are more irritating than painful, but they can cause soreness where they enter the skin. You can minimize discomfort by immobilizing the drains as much as possible, so they don't pull your skin. Pin the plastic loop on top of each drain to

FIGURE 14.1. Fluids from the incision site are collected in surgical drains.

the inside of your robe or to your shirt, belt loop, or waistband to hold it away from the incision and keep it from swinging or catching on furniture. When you shower, pin the drain loops to a long shoelace draped around your neck to keep them from swinging around. Always position drains below your chest incision so they'll drain properly.

Drains are lumpy under clothing. Until they're removed, camouflage is your best fashion defense. Slip on an oversized shirt or sweater and the drains will be hidden from view. Post-mastectomy garments such as the Softee camisole (www.softeeusa .com) have built-in pockets for surgical drains. When your drains come out, you can remove the pockets and have a soft everyday camisole. Another clever garment (designed by a woman

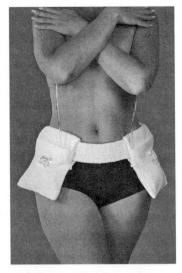

FIGURE 14.2. The Marsupial terry-cloth belt comfortably holds drains in pouches. *Image provided by Tony Cane-Honeysett.*

who has been through mastectomy) is the Marsupial (www.turnerhealth .com), a terrycloth belt with attachable pouches that hold surgical drains (figure 14.2).

Emptying the drains. You should empty the drains and measure the contents twice a day, 12 hours apart, at the same time each day. You may need to do this more frequently if they fill up. (This is a good job for your spouse or partner.) Before you leave the hospital, a nurse will show you how to correctly empty the drains and will provide a measuring cup and a daily log to record the amount of fluid collected.

Here's what you'll do:

1. Wash your hands thoroughly with soap and water before and after handling drains.
2. Unpin the drain from your clothing or remove it from your camisole pouch.
3. Hold the tube with one hand where it enters your skin, and slide the fingers of your other hand down the length of the tube to empty all fluids into the drain bulb.

4. Open the top of the drain bulb and empty the contents into the measuring container. Be sure to squeeze the bulb to empty it completely. Note the color and characteristics of the fluid. Initially it will be bloody, then yellowish, and finally clear. Notify your doctor if the fluid is cloudy, milky, or foul-smelling.

5. Record the amount of fluid on the log provided by the hospital.

6. Flush the fluid down the toilet.

7. Squeeze the empty bulb flat to expel all the air, and close the plug. This creates the suction necessary to remove fluids from the incision. Repin the drain to your clothing or place it back in your pouch.

8. Repeat the process with each drain.

9. Rinse out the measuring container, and wash your hands again.

Keep an eye out for signs of infection in the skin around the drain tube. Call your surgeon if you have any telltale symptoms. Once the level of emptied fluid drops below 30 cc (about 2 tablespoons) in a 24-hour period (for each drain), your surgeon will remove the drains. She'll first snip the suture, then quickly yank the tubing out of your skin. You won't feel any discomfort if you take a big breath and forcibly exhale as she pulls the tube out.

> *Those drains were the worst part of my reconstruction. One wouldn't have been so bad, but I had four: one at each breast and two in my hips. One day the tubing caught on a doorknob as I walked by. It yanked sharply against the incision. That hurt!*   —Kate

Tips for an Easier Recovery

Much of your recovery depends on your own actions. First and foremost, be relentless in taking care of yourself. Until you recover, you can't return to your roles as mom, wife, partner, wage-earner, or caretaker. You have one priority now, and that is to heal. *You* have to be Number One—not the job, not the kids, not anyone else. You can't expect to come home from the hospital and immediately get back up to normal speed. You needn't treat yourself like an invalid. Just don't overdo it.

Getting in and out of bed. Be very careful when you get in and out of bed. Those simple movements we take for granted each morning and night will now be difficult. Think about how you're going to move before you actually do. To get into bed, first sit on the edge and then swing your legs up. Cover your reconstructed breast with one arm and leverage your position with the other. Move up the bed by scooting your behind from side to side until you're reclining against the pillows. To get out of bed after unilateral reconstruction, carefully roll onto your healthy side and use your unaffected arm to leverage yourself into a sitting position. If you've had bilateral reconstruction, use your legs and abdominal muscles to first bring yourself into a sitting position, then swing your legs over the side. Plant your feet on the floor and slowly straighten your knees until you're standing. Entry and exit get trickier if you have an abdominal incision. You'll need someone to help you, while you hold one arm over your chest and the other over your abdomen. If your bedroom is upstairs, consider sleeping on the main floor until you can easily manage the stairs.

The art of sleeping comfortably. Rest and sleep allow your body to direct its resources toward healing, but finding a comfortable position once you get home can be challenging. If you're used to sleeping on your front or side, it will be several weeks before you're able to do that. You need to sleep in a semi-upright position, as you did in the hospital. This keeps fluids from accumulating in your chest and makes getting out of bed easier. This position may feel a bit strange at first. Many women find it more comfortable to sleep in a recliner that is easily repositioned and easier to get in and out of than a bed.

One way to rest comfortably in bed is to make a nest of pillows. First position a firm pillow against the headboard or wall—a body pillow with arm extensions or a sofa cushion works well—then arrange several pillows in front of it to serve as a backrest. Once you're in bed, lean against the pillows behind you. Ask someone to reposition them until you're comfortable. Place pillows under your knees and elevate your surgery-side arm (or both arms if you've had bilateral reconstruction) on additional pillows to take pressure off your chest. If you had a TRAM or DIEP operation, sleep on your back with your head and knees elevated to relieve tension on your abdomen. You might be more comfortable lying flat on your back with your knees together after a TUG or GAP procedure. If you just can't get to sleep or stay asleep, ask your surgeon for a mild sleeping medication.

Sleeping exclusively on your back and spending so much time in bed can give you a backache. Carefully and gently stretch your back to keep it limber and ward off discomfort. Do isometric exercises in bed, first contracting the muscles along the spine, then releasing them in small concentrated movements. Shrug your shoulders and roll your neck gently from side to side. When you're out of bed, stand straight while you flex your spine, as if you're pushing it against a wall, and then pull it back towards you. Do this several times a day.

My husband was afraid of rolling into me and slept in our guest room for six weeks after my reconstruction. It was the only time in our marriage when we slept apart, but it helped. I slept better and he was close enough to hear me if I needed something during the night.   —Karina

Diet and nutrition. It's not unusual to gain weight during recovery. You'll be exercising less and perhaps eating more treats than you normally do, yet now is not the time to diet. Your body will heal faster if you give it the balanced nutrition it needs. Indulge in moderation. Ask friends who provide meals to bring salads or nutritious entrées instead of just cakes, cookies, or other high-fat foods. Enjoy a special treat now and then, but try to eat sensibly and stay hydrated each day.

Listen to your body. Until you're fully recovered, you'll need to rest throughout the day. Don't be afraid to say "not now" if you're not up to a visit or a telephone call. It's good to have time to yourself, to reflect, accept, and just be.

Regain strength, flexibility, and mobility. The therapeutic benefits of exercise have been recognized since ancient times. Exercising moderately for just 30 minutes a day enhances physical and mental well-being. It clears the mind, increases energy, controls weight, and improves overall health. It can help prepare you for surgery, and it's absolutely vital for recovery. When pain and contracting scar tissue impair your range of motion as you heal, restorative movements stimulate circulation and restore flexibility. Regularly performing the right exercises will put you firmly on the road to recovery. Your surgeon will let you know when you should start exercising, usually two to four weeks after surgery, depending on your level of recovery and the type of reconstruction you had. Here are some other helpful resources for cancer survivors and post-surgical patients:

The ACS provides *Essential Exercises for Breast Cancer Survivors*, a booklet of illustrated exercises, divided into four levels of difficulty, to recondition your chest, arms, and shoulders. Call your local ACS office for a copy, or print the exercises and directions from the ACS website (www.cancer.org).

The Lance Armstrong Foundation website describes and illustrates helpful post-mastectomy exercises (www.livestrong.com/article/28314 -post-mastectomy-exercises).

Your YWCA, local hospital, or breast clinic may offer classes designed for women who have had mastectomy.

The Cancer Support Community and LIVESTRONG offer the Cancer Transitions Program (www.cancertransitions.org), which helps patients who have completed treatment in the past 24 months realize the benefits of proper physical activity and nutrition. The program is offered in local groups across the country and online.

If you've had a flap reconstruction, your plastic surgeon will provide a list of additional exercises designed to strengthen and stretch your donor site muscles. Ease carefully into any kind of exercise, skipping any movement that feels too strenuous. It may be helpful to do exercises after a shower, when your muscles are warm and relaxed. The tightness across your chest and in your underarms will improve as you continue your exercise program. Begin cautiously, perform all movements gently, and never stretch or pull to the point of pain. Move smoothly and with awareness. You might need to refrain from weight-bearing and abdominal exercises for up to eight weeks after a TRAM (especially an attached TRAM) or DIEP flap.

Yoga conditions your body before surgery; it's also beneficial once you've recovered sufficiently. Simple restorative poses are best in the beginning, before you progress to more strenuous movements—until you've healed enough, you definitely need to avoid Downward Facing Dog, handstands, and other poses that put pressure on your chest. Ditto with stretches that are too intense for the abdomen or other donor site after flap reconstruction. If you had reconstruction with breast implants, your plastic surgeon may want you to avoid yoga poses that involve the pectoral muscles until your muscles have healed. No matter what exercise or movement you do, if it feels weird or wrong, don't do it. Yoga Bear (www.yogabear.org), a nonprofit organization that offers free yoga classes to cancer survivors, has local studios around the country and also provides short instructive videos online. Breast cancer survivor and yogi Susan Rosen has an easy-to-follow regimen on her video designed especially for breast surgery patients: "Yoga and the Gentle Art of Healing: A Journey of Recovery after Breast Cancer" (www.yogajoyofdelmar.com).

Speak to ten different women who have undergone prophylactic surgeries and you will hear ten distinct stories. Some have wonderful outcomes right away, others struggle for some time; it is plastic surgery after all. Regardless of the outcome or the difficulty, women undergoing surgery and reconstruction will be fine. Our bodies have an amazing ability to heal. —Janet

Seeing Your New Breasts for the First Time

It's not unusual to have conflicting feelings about seeing your new breasts. On one hand, you'll be expectant and hopeful, waiting to see the outcome of several months of planning, surgery, recovery, and waiting. You may feel anxious about what you'll see as you look down at your chest or into a mirror. The reconstruction photos you saw during your research are no longer important, because this is personal. These are your breasts, not someone else's. While most women react positively to reconstruction, some find themselves a bit at odds with their new breasts. At first, your breasts may be bruised and swollen and not look at all the way you'd hoped they would. Don't be surprised if your surgeon proclaims your breasts to be beautiful. Being far more used to this than you are, she's able to see beyond the swelling and redness to visualize the final outcome. Remember that you're a work in progress. This isn't what you'll look like several months or a year from now, when you're fully healed and your scars have faded. You've suffered a very personal loss. Give yourself time to come to grips with it and grieve for it, if that feels right. The recovery process is temporary. Hang in there and know that the worst is behind you.

When I first saw my reconstructed breasts, I burst into tears. They were horrible! My doctor smiled and said my two little ugly ducklings would grow up to be beautiful swans, and he was right. Nine months later, when I look at my breasts now it is hard to imagine they had such an ugly beginning.
—Holly

CHAPTER FIFTEEN

Dealing with Problems

Obstacles don't have to stop you. If you run into a wall, don't turn around and give up. Figure out how to climb it, go through it, or work around it. —MICHAEL JORDAN

All surgery has a potential for complications, and breast reconstruction is no exception. Even though serious problems are uncommon, there is always the risk of infection, a negative reaction to anesthesia, or an unsatisfactory cosmetic result. When problems linger beyond recovery or become severe, corrective steps can and should be taken. You don't have to live with these problems, and in most cases they can be resolved satisfactorily during revision surgery or in a minor procedure in your surgeon's office. Chapters 6 through 9 discuss problems that are specific to expander, implant, or flap reconstruction. Other complications that may occur as a result of mastectomy or reconstruction are explained in this chapter.

Inherent Surgical Risks

Any surgery with general anesthesia carries risks for complications; some are more common than others. Although most women experience none of these, one or more problems may develop after your mastectomy or reconstruction.

Bleeding. Excessive bleeding is unlikely after surgery, particularly when incisions are made with electrocautery tools, which use high-voltage electrical current to cut through soft tissue and seal off blood vessels. Still, it's important to heed your surgeon's caution to discontinue using vitamins, herbs, and medicines that thin the blood. Your doctor will advise you when you should stop taking them before your surgery, and when you can begin taking them again. A damaged blood vessel may leak into the surrounding tissue, forming a *hematoma*: the greater the leakage, the larger the hematoma. Symptoms include pain or a feeling of fullness at the leakage site; the skin may appear dark, as though it's bruised. Your surgeon will want to monitor any hematoma closely, because if it grows too large, it may compress tissues and prevent oxygen from reaching the skin, potentially causing infection, a wound that opens or leaks fluid or blood, and necrosis. A hematoma that isn't *resorbed* (assimilated back into the body) may require surgery to reopen the incision, drain the pooled blood, and reseal the blood vessel. You're at higher risk for excessive bleeding or hematoma if you have a bleeding disorder or hypertension. Hematomas can develop within hours of surgery or even months later if too much pressure is put on the breast— you fall down, you're elbowed in a crowd, or your partner engages in over-zealous squeezing of your new breast.

Seroma. A seroma is similar to a hematoma but involves an accumulation of clear fluid (rather than blood) that leaks from blood vessels, even when compression garments and surgical drains are used. Seromas can be quite small or large enough to cause significant swelling—you may even hear fluid sloshing when you move. These symptoms may be accompanied by pain and skin discoloration, warmth, or redness. Left untreated, seromas can harden and become infected, and then you'll need antibiotics. If the excess fluid isn't eventually resorbed, your surgeon may need to drain the site with a needle or insert another surgical drain for a few days. If the problem area grows large enough to restrict oxygen supply to the tissue, it may require surgical repair.

Infection. Skin is the body's natural barrier to infection; anytime the skin is opened, infection has an opportunity to sneak in. Precautionary procedures, such as maintaining a sterile operating environment, cleansing incision sites with antibacterial wash, and dispensing antibiotics through your IV, help protect you during your surgery. You're more susceptible to infection if you smoke, are obese, have diabetes, are receiving chemotherapy, or have had previous breast radiation. Infection is of particular concern when you have tissue expanders or implants. Like all types of implants used in the body, expanders and breast implants can become contaminated by bacteria in the bloodstream or through an infection in the body, and then capsular contracture may develop. For this reason, some plastic surgeons suggest their implant patients take antibiotics preventively before any subsequent invasive procedures, including colonoscopy, cosmetic surgery, and even dental work, including teeth cleaning. Surgeons have no standard guidelines and no consensus about this, and their opinions on the matter differ.

Treating a lingering infection usually involves removing the implant and *debriding* (removing unhealthy tissue from) the pocket to promote healing, followed by a course of antibiotics. If the implant is removed, a new one can be placed several months later. Contact your surgeon immediately if you develop signs of infection.

> *My plastic surgeon initially planned to fill the tissue expanders a little after my mastectomy so I wouldn't be completely flat when I woke up. When she attempted to fill them, the breast skin on the right side began to die, so she removed the saline on that side. A week later, I had my first debridement surgery, but the incision popped open again the following week. After another debridement, the incision stayed closed, but my back, stomach, and scar line became red. My entire breast was also red and swollen. I had a cellulitis infection and needed two strong antibiotics for ten days. Then fluid began to leak from my scar, and the surgeon had to remove the expander. Now my left expander is filled to where I want it, and I'm waiting to have a latissimus dorsi flap with implant reconstruction to replace the other expander that was removed.* —Marti

Delayed wound healing. Some individuals take longer to heal than others, particularly when a weakened immune system or chronic health problem becomes an issue and leads to *delayed wound healing*. Diabetics, for instance, may heal more slowly from surgery than non-diabetics. Infection slows the healing process, so take every precaution to prevent it: keep the area around your incisions scrupulously clean and wash your hands frequently.

Your body expends copious amounts of energy during the healing process; you can promote healing by eating a variety of nutritious foods each day. Include sufficient protein and vitamins A and C, and be sure to eat enough calories. If you don't have much of an appetite as you recover, eat several nutrition-dense meals throughout the day, rather than just two or three larger meals.

Necrosis. Breast skin is fragile after mastectomy. If it's exceptionally thin after the breast tissue is cut away or is handled too roughly, it may die. The same result may occur if the breast surgeon severs too many blood vessels that feed the skin or uses electrocautery too aggressively and burns the inside of the skin, which may then blister and die. Infrequently, a small amount of fat in the flap or surrounding an implant turns dark or hardens because it doesn't get enough blood. Your surgeon needs to know about this right away. Depending on the extent of the problem, he may advise a wait-and-see approach or recommend massage for several weeks to soften the area. If a small area of necrosis doesn't shrink on its own, it can be surgically removed. A more serious, although rare, problem is the death of an entire tissue flap because the supplying blood vessels are blocked—the flap must be removed, and unless you prefer to be flat, a new procedure (with an implant or another flap) is required to again rebuild the breast. Necrosis develops more frequently in smokers, women with circulatory problems, and those who have had previous lumpectomy and radiation.[1]

My right DIEP reconstruction was beautiful; my left side was less coopera-tive due to a compromised blood supply. After a lengthy operation and another surgery the following day to try to connect the flap artery to a blood vessel in my underarm, my plastic surgeon said we'd have to wait and see how my left breast fared. After eight weeks, some of the tissue lived and some did not. Compared to my natural-looking right breast, my left breast was small, hard, and lumpy; they were far from a matching set. During an outpatient surgery, the dead flap tissue was cut away and I was fitted with an expander. I am still waiting for my filled expander to rest before exchanging it for an implant. Though I never thought I'd focus so much attention and time on my boobs, I realize that in the big picture, fifteen months of surgeries, healing, and waiting is really not long at all. I waited longer for my youngest to sleep through the night when he was a baby!
                                                                    —Jenni

Lingering Pain

Even though most post-reconstruction discomfort gradually disappears, some women experience pain or muscle spasms after their incisions have healed. There's a big difference between ordinary discomfort as healing progresses and subsequent chronic or intense pain. And though you may be content to live with cosmetic flaws, you should always seek help for unrelenting pain. Aside from interfering with your well-being, it slows the immune system's ability to fight off disease and infection. Persistent pain can be caused by a damaged nerve, a hematoma or seroma, chemotherapy, or radiation treatment. Sometimes, lack of appropriate reconditioning is the cause. A cycle of pain may continue, for example, when you don't properly rehabilitate your arm and shoulder after surgery: it hurts, you don't use it, it gets worse.

About half of women who have axillary lymph node dissection, lumpectomy, or mastectomy develop intermittent or persistent chronic pain, most likely caused by severing or damaging the intercostobrachial nerves that provide sensation to the shoulder and upper arm.[2] This *intercostobrachial neuralgia (ICN)*, which includes *post-mastectomy pain syndrome*, is rarely discussed as a potential risk of breast surgery. It isn't clearly defined or well studied, and regrettably, it's not fully understood or acknowledged. Physicians often assume the pain is simply a residual side effect of mastectomy. In many cases, burning or tingling in the arm, shoulder, or chest wall can be debilitating, disrupting sleep and quality of life. ICN occurs more frequently in women under age 40 and in those who have had breast radiation therapy.

If you experience strong and unrelenting pain, you may need a CT scan to try to pinpoint the cause. Depending on the severity of the pain, treatment may include non-steroidal anti-inflammatory drugs (NSAIDs), including aspirin, ibuprofen, and naproxen; corticosteroid injections; or nerve medications. A mild antidepressant sometimes provides relief. Your doctor can also administer a series of anesthetic injections to block sensory nerve paths. Physical therapy and acupuncture can help, as does regular exercise, which prompts your body to release endorphins, chemicals that block pain signals to the brain. It may take a process of trial and error to find a solution that works. If pain persists, ask for a referral to a pain specialist, preferably someone who has experience identifying and treating ICN.

Lymphedema

Women who have lymph nodes removed or have radiation therapy have a lifetime risk of lymphedema—the risk is higher if you have nodes removed *and* radiation therapy, and lower if you have a sentinel node biopsy. There's no way to predict who will develop lymphedema and who won't. It may appear soon after lumpectomy or mastectomy, or months or even years later. The affected arm may feel heavy, tight, or numb. Swelling in the arm may be almost unnoticeable, like fluid retention during your menstrual period. In extreme cases, the arm becomes enlarged from shoulder to fingertips. Contact your doctor at the first sign of swelling, even mild swelling, in your arm or chest after breast surgery. Lymphedema is chronic and incurable. When treated early, however, it can be controlled with compression sleeves, special exercises, and therapeutic massage. The National Lymphedema Network (www.lymphnet.org) provides information and support for this condition.

Be very protective of the affected arm. Keep it scrupulously clean to avoid infection, and protect it from burns, cuts, and other injuries. Injections, blood samples, or blood pressure readings should always be taken from your unaffected arm. Historically, women with lymphedema were advised to avoid lifting with the affected arm, but research shows that twice-weekly gentle weight lifting increases strength and decreases symptoms.[3] If you have lymphedema, talk to your doctor before you begin any strength training regimen for your affected arm. Then meet with a fitness trainer who has training in the specific weight-lifting regimen for lymphedema, or ask your local YMCA about the LIVESTRONG program for cancer survivors, which uses the same protocol.

Surgical approaches to lymphedema are also being studied. *Axillary reverse mapping* is a promising procedure that uses a blue dye to identify underarm nodes, allowing surgeons to remove nodes that drain the breast and preserve nodes that drain the arm.[4] *Vascularized lymph node transfer* is a microsurgical approach for individuals who don't respond to conventional treatment.[5] It replaces the removed lymph nodes with healthy nodes, which then pick up the job of draining lymphatic fluids. Used in Europe and China with some success, vascularized lymph node transfer is gaining interest in the United States, primarily as a companion surgery to microsurgical abdominal breast reconstruction. While the flap incision is open, lymph nodes are harvested from the donor site and transplanted to the underarm. More surgeons may become trained to offer this surgery—and health care insurers may agree to cover it—if clinical trials show it's safe and effective and doesn't remedy lymphedema at one location only to have it develop at the donor site.

> *My arm, hand, and fingers began to swell right after my mastectomy. I couldn't bend my wrist or straighten my arm all the way, and it throbbed constantly. It was impossible to hold or carry my baby. I suffered for several months until my doctor sent me to a physical therapist who taught my husband how to do a special massage. We've made this a part of our daily routine. I feel better and my husband is happy he can do something to help. The lymphedema is still there; at least it's manageable now.*   —Skye

Cosmetic Do-Overs

It would be wonderful if every patient emerged from the operating room with superb results. The reality is that most breast reconstruction requires revision. It's part and parcel of the reconstruction process, and some remedies are easier than others. A minor outpatient procedure may be all that is needed to correct indentations in the breast, a dog ear at the end of a scar, or other minimal cosmetic flaws that mar an otherwise fine breast. Lingering complications of larger proportions may require additional revision surgery. If your breast is too big, it can be reduced. If your implant is too small, it can be replaced with one that is larger. A breast can be lifted if it's too low or dropped if it's too high. Displeased with the way your belly button was stretched after your abdominal flap? Your surgeon can improve this, too. Revision surgery often takes care of problems or makes them more acceptable; some are impossible to fix.

The best defense is a good offense. While you can't eliminate all possibility of post-recovery complications, taking a few precautions beforehand will help minimize the chance that you'll develop post-op problems and cosmetic flaws.

Choose the best surgeon you can find. Chapter 17 shows you how.

Manage your expectations. Go into surgery with realistic expectations of your outcome, so you won't be surprised when your expanding breast sits too high on your chest or when it doesn't exactly match the opposite side. If you decide to proceed with implant reconstruction even though your surgeon advises that your post-radiation skin is too thin, understand that you have a good chance of developing complications.

Give yourself adequate time to heal. While it's normal to feel impatient, try not to jump to conclusions before you're fully healed, because many problems eventually resolve on their own. Reconstructed breasts improve over time; your flap or implant reconstruction will look considerably better after a year than it does just two or three months after your initial operation. What is now a misshapen or asymmetrical breast may be fine once the swelling disappears and it drops into its final position; however, it may take a year or more for scars to fade.

Decide what's acceptable and what's not. We are our own harshest critics. Subtle flaws in your breast that are all but invisible to your partner may be objectionable to you. (It's interesting to note that many women who are somewhat unsatisfied with their reconstructed breasts say their husband or partner thinks they're just fine.) You might decide you can live with the tiny bulge in your new breast or the wide scar on your abdomen, or you might consider these unacceptable. After recovery, perhaps you'll feel that you just can't face yet another procedure and you're willing to accept what you have as good enough. Or you may want to keep trying to correct flaws that are irksome to you.

Understand what can be changed and accept what cannot. When all is said and done, some problems cannot be fixed. Surgeons can't restore full sensation or eliminate scars, and they may not be able to give you two identical breasts, especially if you've had radiation therapy. Revision surgery may improve the look of your breast; it still may not get it as close to perfect as you'd hoped. At some point, you must accept that your reconstruction is as good as it can be.

Take action. There's no need to suffer in silence. Acknowledging a problem is the first step in treating it. While the thought of additional appointments, procedures, and even minor recovery may be unsettling, discuss your dissatisfaction with your surgeon. He's probably seen and heard it all before, and he can determine whether the problem is likely to run its course or deserves additional attention. If your surgeon approached the initial reconstructive process enthusiastically but isn't so keen about handling problems after the fact, look for another opinion if you're unhappy with his response to your concerns.

Address lumps, bumps, and bulges. Although a lump is the last thing a cancer patient wants to find in her new breast, it's not uncommon to find a small lump in a reconstructed breast, particularly after flap reconstruction or a fat graft. Discovering a hard spot can be unnerving, especially if you've already been through the breast cancer experience; most often, it's a bit of fat that has hardened or died. A glob of fat may poke up under the skin or along the edge of the flap. Some patients develop suture *granulomas*, scar tissue that forms around the internal sutures used to close your incisions. Most sutures used for mastectomy and reconstruction are absorbable, although your body may have different ideas about that. It will react to any foreign material, even tiny sutures. You may notice a "spitting suture" where your body pushes a stitch out through the skin. Your surgeon may advise you to massage the area for a few weeks to see whether the sutures will be absorbed by your body, or he may aspirate the lump with a needle to determine the cause. If the lump doesn't soften on its own in a few months, it can be surgically removed or liposuctioned away.

> *Several months after my TRAM, I developed what I called my third boob.*
> *It was this A-cup size lump sticking out above my waistline. My doctor*
> *said it was the result of tunneling the flap up under the skin. It did finally*
> *shrink, but it took almost a year.*   —B.J.

Fixes with Fat

Surgeons have successfully used *fat grafting* (also called *lipofilling*) for years to correct cosmetic defects of the face, hands, and other parts of the body. Fat taken from your own body and injected into your new breast can be used to improve dimples, dents, wrinkles, and other small imperfections. It can't, however, just be scooped from your hips and plopped directly onto your breast. (A fat graft isn't the same as a tissue flap that is used to reconstruct a breast after mastectomy: a fat graft depends on blood and nutrients in the chest, while a tissue flap has its own blood supply.) While you're under local or general anesthesia, fat is liposuctioned from your abdomen, thigh, hip, or wherever you have it to spare. (Unless your fatty deposits are obvious, your surgeon can do a quick pinch test to determine where sufficient fat lies beneath the skin.) It is then liquified, purified, and injected into the breast defect. The injected fat connects to blood vessels in the new breast, much like a skin graft does. That's why fat injections are limited to small areas of the breast: an adequate blood supply can't reach all areas of a large blob of fat. It's hard to predict how much fat will take hold in the breast and how much will be resorbed. If necessary, the process can be repeated in three to six months. Although lipofilling can improve the appearance of your reconstructed breasts, it's generally considered a poor idea to use flap surgery to recreate an undersized breast, with the intention of later using fat injections to "pump" it up to the desired size. Ever-improving procedures are being studied to increase the level of fat that stays in the breast after lipofilling.

One concern about fat grafting has been that stem cells in transplanted fat might trigger new cancer growth. Initial studies have found this concern to be unfounded. A clinical study in Europe (where fat grafting is used more frequently than in the United States) concluded that after an average of 4.6 years, women who had lipofilling after lumpectomy had no greater risk of recurrence than those who did not have the procedure.[6] While these results are encouraging, longer term follow-up research is needed.

Fat added to the breast can develop palpable pearl-sized lumps about a year after surgery. While this isn't a cancer recurrence or cause for alarm, it can be anxiety provoking and should be brought to your surgeon's attention.

Fat Injections for Breast Reconstruction

FRANK J. DELLACROCE, MD, FACS

Re-injecting liquid fat collected during liposuction to improve soft tissue volume problems is a technique that has waxed and waned in popularity for many decades. Only recently has fat injection regained attention as a tool to help improve volume and contour problems left behind after breast reconstruction with an implant or flap procedure. No controlled, long-term studies have been performed, so independent reports of reliability, consistent take of the fat, or amount of fat that can be expected to survive are variable, with little objective data to back them up. There is consensus, however, that fat injection has a place in breast reconstruction, that it is relatively safe, and that it is useful for small contour or volume problems that are otherwise difficult to correct. Outcomes are technique dependent: gentle handling of the fat and applying small droplets in many different locations helps maximize fat survival. Survival of injected fat is difficult to predict and control, and repeat injections are commonly needed. Fifty percent take of the fat is respectable—in many cases it will be less. Previous radiation of tissues may adversely affect success rates. Caution should be exercised when choosing fat injection, since the associated suctioning may eliminate the option for later flap reconstruction if implants or other means of reconstruction fall short of expectations.

Improving Scars

Scarring is a natural part of the body's healing process and an unavoidable side effect of surgery. Tissue scars when the *epidermis*, or outer layer of skin, is damaged—when you badly burn your finger or get a deep cut, for example. When the *dermis*, the thick tissue beneath the epidermis, is affected—as when a surgical incision is made—the body produces a connective tissue protein called *collagen* to fill in the gaps. It's the body's version of spackle that forms the scar. Scars look different from the rest of your skin because collagen looks different. It has no sweat glands or pores. When too much collagen is produced, the result is a thicker, more prominent scar.

Why does your friend's TRAM scar look so much better than yours? The appearance of a scar is determined by a person's age and genetics, the depth of the wound, and how the incision and underlying tissues are sewn together. If you smoke or have poor circulation, inhibited blood flow at the incision site may make for a more obvious scar. Any scars you have from previous surgeries or wounds are a good indication of how your reconstruction scar will heal.

Reconstruction scars are red, angry looking, and hard to ignore after surgery. They fade to pink after two to three months, as collagen and new blood vessels heal the incisions. Mastectomy and reconstruction scars never disappear, but most fade within a year or two after surgery; in another year or so, they're just thin white lines. Others may remain deeply pigmented, bumpy, or raised. What can you do to minimize scars? Other than silicone sheeting or gel that improves excessive scarring, no well-studied evidence shows that any topical treatment makes a significant improvement. Here are a few suggestions to promote healing and make your scars smoother, flatter, and less noticeable.

- Leave the wound alone. Try not to fuss with your incision or pick at the steri-tape or surgical glue that compress the edges of the wound together to keep the scar line as thin as possible.
- Moisturize. As soon as your incisions close and your surgeon approves, apply aloe vera, cocoa butter, or mineral oil to the wound; a moist wound heals better than a dry wound. Never moisturize a fresh incision, which may invite infection and make the scar worse. Wait until it's fully healed. Read labels to avoid products that include preservatives, fragrance, and alcohol, which dries the skin. Vitamin E oil may be an adequate moisturizer; no solid evidence shows that it improves scarring.
- Massage the scar line. As you rub in lotion or cream, massage the scar with your fingertips to stretch and break down fibers beneath the skin. Apply pressure along the length of the scar, then across it. Massage deeply, but not to the point of pain. Roll the scar between your fingers each day to keep the tissue soft.
- Give your body adequate vitamin C and zinc. Both aid in wound healing. Taking a good multivitamin that includes both should do the trick, or add several servings of citrus, green leafy vegetables, and foods that are high in protein to your daily diet.
- Protect your scars from ultraviolet light. Scars may darken and become hard if exposed to sunlight or tanning beds during the first year after surgery. Even indirect sun exposure can adversely affect their appearance. Apply a sunblock of SPF 20 or higher, with UVA and UVB protection, at least 20 minutes before you go outside, and repeat frequently.
- Apply a scar management product. Over-the-counter products won't eliminate scars, but they might help to improve their appearance. You must use them consistently—10 to 18 hours a day for several

months—for them to have an effect. You might also consider using a silicone or hydrogel sheet to improve redness and flatten raised areas.

Some women develop large *hypertrophic scars* that rise above the level of the surrounding skin and remain painful or tender. *Keloids* are thick scars that spread into the skin around the incision. Although anyone can develop keloids, they're more common in dark-skinned women. (If other family members develop keloids, you're more likely to have them as well.) Let your surgeon know if you're prone to problem scarring, so he can use a different type of suture, which may help. The International Advisory Panel on Scar Management recommends applying silicone gel sheeting as soon as an incision is healed to prevent hypertrophic scars and keloids—you'll need to wear the product for 12 to 24 hours each day for several months to achieve the best results.

If all else fails, ask your surgeon or dermatologist about the following scar-minimizing treatments:

- injecting cortisone or a steroid into the scar to reduce collagen production and temporarily soften the tissue
- applying topical aspirin and salicylic acid
- surgically revising the scar by cutting away the hard tissue and re-suturing the incision; it doesn't guarantee that your new scar will be better—hypertrophic and keloidal scars recur about half the time—though it may be worth a try if your scars are bothersome
- treatment with a fractional carbon dioxide (CO_2) laser

My scar had a big pucker right in the front of my breast. In about 20 minutes, my surgeon reopened the incision, cut away the scar tissue, and sewed it back up. It felt tight for a few weeks, and then it healed and looked better than before.   *—Donna*

My mastectomy scar is horrible and thick. Even though my doctor revised it, three years later, it's still pretty bad. I knew that was a possibility because I've never scarred well, even from minor cuts. My doctor said it's as good as it's going to get.   *—Jean*

CHAPTER SIXTEEN

Life after Reconstruction

Cancer was a gift that helped me grow. —RUDOLPH GIULIANI

At last. After months of doctors' appointments, surgeries, and recovery, your reconstruction journey is over. Your new breasts are in place, and you're ready to move on. You may feel a wonderful sense of closure as you leave your plastic surgeon's office for the last time. Or you might experience sadness or depression, particularly if you've come to regard your surgeon as a trusted friend. This isn't unusual. You've spent a lot of time together during your reconstruction, and now your emotional umbilical cord is about to be severed. Your life is finally getting back to normal.

Adjusting to the New You

It's often said that cancer is a journey. Sometimes we don't realize that until we reach the end of the process and look back. If only hindsight had arrived a little sooner! If you can view reconstruction that way—as an odyssey with an outcome—you'll fare better. When you're uncomfortable, uneasy, or fed up with the reconstruction ordeal, remember it isn't a life sentence. It's a finite experience with a beginning, middle, and end. You won't ever forget your mastectomy and reconstruction, but eventually, personal and professional priorities that were shelved during the process will be restored in your life, and your surgeries and recovery will be a distant memory. Your emotional and physical scars will heal, and you'll return to a life without surgeons, weird sleeping positions, or checking your breasts throughout the day. You'll be just fine.

It takes time to get used to the idea of losing a breast. Sometimes it takes a lot of tears, too. Your new breasts will be very different from your natural breasts, and that takes some getting used to as well, even if they look the same. Most of us can't simply flick an emotional switch and go seamlessly from being patients to being disease-free women. If you're nagged by depression that you just can't seem to shake, even when your reconstruction is completed, consider the following.

- Put your breast cancer and reconstruction in perspective. It's a bit of a cliché, but cancer does change your perspective. Treatment and reconstruction offer positives for those who are open to them. Learn—or re-learn—to appreciate life and all it offers. Separate the nickel-and-dime issues, like getting stuck in traffic or burning the toast, from the truly serious.
- Reprioritize. Actor Michael J. Fox once said, "Illness forces you to get rid of the clutter in your life to make room for the priorities." He was referring to his own fight against Parkinson's disease, but his words ring true for any life-altering experience. Figure out what's important in your life and move those things to the top of your priority list. Don't feel guilty about items that sink to the bottom and don't get done.
- Don't hide from your feelings. Grief and angst come in all sizes. Some women are emotionally strong, taking mastectomy and reconstruction in their stride with a Zen-like approach or an "I don't have time for this" attitude. Others find it impossible to regain any sense of the normal. It's okay—and healthy—to react in the way that's natural for you. At some point, though, you'll get tired of being angry, tired of being sad, and tired of having your life put on hold. The best possible therapy is to acknowledge your feelings and let 'em rip. Then dust off your emotional self and move forward.
- Turn off the negative self-talk. It happens to the best of us: sooner or later those dark thoughts creep into our consciousness. When you catch yourself thinking negatively, replace those thoughts with positive affirmations.
- Focus on your post-reconstruction life. Appreciate the loss you've suffered from mastectomy, but also consider the control you've gained over breast cancer.
- Create an outlet for your emotions. Don't get caught in a downward spiral of adverse emotions. Deal with your feelings before they begin controlling your life. Talk to your partner, a trusted friend or family

member, a member of the clergy, or a local support group. Writing is also therapeutic. Try your hand at poetry or journaling, letting your thoughts flow freely and uncensored onto the paper or computer screen.

- Ask for help. If negative thoughts persist and become more than a temporary funk, consider seeing a mental health professional who can help you resolve troubling issues.

Understand that friends mean well. Your friends will want the best for you, even when it doesn't seem that way. While most people you know will be nothing but supportive, some people have a hard time dealing with illness, surgery, or recovery. Friends may not be able to look you in the eye without crying. You may find yourself comforting them, instead of the other way around. Others may be embarrassed or may struggle for the right thing to say. Some may be unable to accept the fact that you're fine, even after your recovery. They'll continue to view you as a victim, even long after you're back to your normal routine. Each time they see you, they'll ask in a soft, sad voice, "How are you?" Don't be surprised if some folks can't seem to draw their eyes away from your chest. Many are quite curious about mastectomy and reconstruction; when they realize they're talking to your chest, they may become terribly embarrassed. They're all trying to help, in their own way. Just take a deep breath and realize they mean no harm.

Remember to laugh. Mastectomy and reconstruction certainly aren't funny, but we can always find humor if we look hard enough. Laughter is powerful medicine. It releases endorphins, sending feel-good messages from the brain throughout the body. Studies suggest that laughter boosts the immune system and reduces pain. One little chuckle or a rollicking belly laugh releases a lot of tension. Ever noticed how quickly kids rebound from sadness? It may have everything to do with laughter—children laugh about 400 times a day; adults, just 25. Find ways to laugh each day. The Cancer Club (www.cancerclub.com) has books, newsletters, and other items that will tickle your funny bone and help you see the lighter side of treatment and reconstruction. Or learn about Laughter Yoga (www.laughter yoga.org), a combination of exercises, deep breathing, and relaxation techniques that is said to combat stress and anxiety.

Mend your mind, body, and spirit. You've beaten cancer and completed reconstruction. Now what? Now you experience the sweet relief of returning to your pre-diagnosis life, before the tests and treatments began. Perhaps, like many breast cancer survivors, you feel a new lease on life, one that compels you to find a fresh balance between physical, emotional, and spiritual health. You may feel the need to take better care of your body, not because anything you did caused your breast cancer, but because living with the disease gives us such a profound gratitude for the bodies we have. For some, it's cause to reassess or reaffirm beliefs. Perhaps you have a renewed conviction to travel, change jobs, help others, or do all those things you've always wanted to do but had to put on the back burner when life got in the way. It's good to look back and reflect. It's better to look forward and embrace the future.

Your turn to share. If you're inclined to share what you've learned from your breast cancer experience, you can help other women who are facing those same mastectomy and reconstruction issues you now have behind you. They want to know more about breast cancer treatment, post-mastectomy options, and recovery. Whether you spend an occasional hour or get involved full-time, there are plenty of opportunities to donate your time, money, and insight.

- Let your oncologist and plastic surgeon know that you're happy to speak with other patients who have questions. Many women will welcome your insight as they consider their post-mastectomy choices and wonder what reconstruction is like.
- Become a Reach to Recovery volunteer for the American Cancer Society.
- Speak to women at your local breast cancer center or support group.
- Donate or raise money for your local breast cancer organization. There are hundreds, if not thousands, of local fundraisers for breast cancer each year across the country. You'll find all kinds of worthwhile opportunities to raise funds for the cause. Call your local ACS office or search the Internet for "breast cancer charity" to find ways to make a difference.
- If you tested positive for a BRCA gene mutation, consider volunteering or becoming a FORCE outreach coordinator.

Back to Work

Returning to work is a giant step on the road back to normal. The workplace can be a positive and caring environment, depending on how close you are to your co-workers and how much they know about why you've been away. If your workplace is a source of stress and uneasiness, take time to consider how you'll deal with it before you return. You may need to ease back into the work routine, especially if the pressures and pace of an entire day are too taxing. It all depends on the extent of your recovery and the nature of your job: you'll be able to return to an administrative job sooner than to a job as police officer or daycare center operator. Perhaps you can work flex hours or part-time until you're back up to speed. If you still feel mentally or physically fatigued, you may need more time to recuperate.

Your relationship with your co-workers will dictate how much you do or don't tell them about your treatment and reconstruction. Many women consider their co-workers as extended family; others prefer not to draw attention to themselves or be treated differently. If you would rather keep your experience private, when someone asks why you were away, you can simply say it was for health reasons or a family issue, or something similar.

Dating, Intimacy, and Sex

Your medical team gives you information about what to expect before and after surgery, but usually, no one explains about how it might affect your intimate relationship with your husband, partner, or boyfriend. Whether you're single or married, you may worry about how your reconstructed breast will affect your romantic involvements. After months of treatment, surgeries, and recovery you may feel disconnected from physical pleasure, and intimacy may feel awkward. Lingering effects of cancer treatment can also take a toll on intimacy, long after your stitches dissolve and your incisions heal. It can take time, effort, and patience to resolve these issues and get your love life back on track. Sharing the experience is important to your relationship and will make things easier for both of you.

Lost breast sensation takes some getting used to, particularly if your breasts used to play a starring role in the bedroom. You don't have to give up the pleasure of your breasts, but you may need to redefine how you go about it. Even though your reduced sensation may be disappointing, you can still enjoy your partner's touch if you concentrate on areas that still provide pleasure. Explore the "new girls" together, guiding his fingertips over them and directing his attention to the areas where you can feel his touch, instead of where you don't.

Although you're the one who goes through reconstruction and recovery, your experience affects your partner as well. You may be perfectly comfortable in your post-mastectomy body and eagerly slip back into the closeness you experienced before your mastectomy and reconstruction. For some women, it's not that easy. With your reconstruction behind you, your partner may assume you'll pick up your relationship where you left off, but it isn't always easy to emotionally just snap out of it. Open communication paves the way for you and your partner to be more comfortable with your new breasts. Express your feelings and encourage your partner to do the same. It may be difficult to talk about your feelings, but it's important to explain how you feel and what you want. Ask for patience if you need more time to achieve arousal, and try telling your partner what feels good and what doesn't, rather than what he's doing wrong. Discuss together how you can change your sexual repertoire (if you need to) to satisfy you both. Try not to assume that your partner perceives you as undesirable if he doesn't initiate intimacy; he may simply be afraid to hurt you or may feel rejected, particularly if you're emotionally distant. He'll probably take his cues from your own attitude and comfort level with your new breasts. If you're comfortable seeing and touching them, your partner probably will be too.

> My husband kept ignoring my reconstructed breast. I couldn't feel much there, but emotionally, it was important to me to include it in our lovemaking. When I mentioned this to him he said he was afraid he would hurt me. After we talked about it, we both felt relieved, like a huge barrier between us had been broken down.   —Alma

Take your time. You've been through a lot. You may be eager to get your love life back to normal, or you may need more time to restore your sexual health. Allow yourself a period of adjustment to get back in the groove.

Take it slowly if you feel shy, uncomfortable, or apprehensive. Rekindle your romantic relationship and let it develop on its own. Spend time alone together, just being affectionate and doing the things you love to do. When you don't feel "in the mood," concentrate on just enjoying each other's company. Hold hands as you go for a walk. Start and end each day with a hug. Make time to share a soothing bath or a romantic dinner. Kiss and cuddle before you progress to the main event. Work toward being comfortable with the new you and let Nature take its course.

If you feel uneasy when you're undressed, wear lingerie or turn off the lights until you become more comfortable with your new breast. Progress at your own pace. Remember, the brain is the most powerful sexual organ we have. You're still very much a woman. Intellectually, you probably know you're still much more than the sum total of your breasts, but it may take a while to believe it. If you continue to feel uncomfortable with intimacy, consider joining a support group or seeking professional guidance; talking with an intimacy expert may be all the help you need to get back to a satisfying relationship. Let yourself heal, grieve your loss, and deal with the aftermath of your cancer and mastectomy. If you can't seem to shake negative thoughts or you feel depressed beyond your control, talk to your doctor or see a therapist about medications that can lift your mood without affecting your libido.

When your partner has a problem. If your spouse or partner has been supportive throughout your mastectomy and reconstruction, you are truly blessed. Most women find their partners to be a constant source of reassurance, loving them for who they are instead of what's on their chest. If the two of you previously shared a strong bond, your relationship is more likely to weather the stress and trauma of mastectomy and reconstruction. If your relationship was weak, your treatment and reconstruction can bring you closer together—or drive you farther apart. Some partners are scared silly by the thought of cancer and surgery, but hesitant to discuss their feelings. Others may react with denial, refusing to acknowledge your cancer and reconstruction. Some—hopefully few—may wonder what the big deal is if you're able to have your breast recreated. Early on, ask your partner to accompany you to doctors' visits, participate fully in your reconstruction research, and support you during recovery.

New relationships. Dating presents an interesting dilemma. When and what do you tell your partner-to-be? "Nice to meet you. My left breast came from my belly" or "I'm finally getting my nipples done tomorrow!" may be a bit much when you're introduced. When should you speak up and how much should you say? There is probably no single right answer to these questions. The best approach is to rely on your instinct to know when the time is right. If you and your date happen to be talking about his mother's struggle with breast cancer, it might be a logical time to share your own experience. In other cases, it may not come up until it's becoming very clear that your relationship is heading to the bedroom. Your own comfort with the topic and how you feel about the other person will dictate when you talk about your reconstruction and how much you say. That might be on your first date, when you're getting to know each other, or it might be later in your relationship.

Surveillance after Mastectomy

Whether your breast was removed prophylactically or because of breast cancer, you've reduced your future risk significantly. It's wise to remain vigilant, but you needn't live your life in fear. Recurrence is unlikely after mastectomy, but leftover cancer cells can form a small lump under the skin, near the mastectomy scar, or in what little breast tissue remains. Some women develop a recurrence in the chest muscle, but that's even more uncommon. A small malignancy in the scar or skin can usually be removed without disturbing the implant or the reconstructed flap; it may also require radiation if you haven't already had it on that side of your chest. Excising a larger tumor may require removing the implant or part of the flap. Alert your surgeon immediately if you find a suspicious area or lump in your reconstructed breast, so he can order whatever tests are necessary to determine whether it is a calcification, a fragment of dead tissue, or a recurrence.

Monitor your reconstructed breast. The ACS recommends that "women who have had total, modified radical, or radical mastectomy for breast cancer need no further routine screening mammograms of the affected side (or sides, if both breasts are removed)." This recommendation makes sense, because most all of your breast tissue has been removed. Some surgeons recommend that women have a baseline mammogram or MRI after reconstruction, so that any unusual area that develops can be scanned and compared. Continued mammograms are advised if you've had a subcutaneous mastectomy (an early type of nipple-sparing mastectomy that left breast tissue at the base of the nipple and is no longer performed). If you have silicone implant reconstruction, the FDA recommends you have an MRI after three years and every two years thereafter, to detect any rupture.

It's wise to continue examining your own breasts each month and to have regular professional examinations as recommended by your oncologist. If a medical professional has never shown you how to do a breast self-exam correctly, ask your doctor or nurse to demonstrate. Or see the instructive video at the Susan G. Komen Breast Cancer Foundation's website (www .komen.org/bse). Do your exam about the same time each month, preferably 7 to 10 days after the first day of your menstrual period (or any time during the month if you no longer have periods). Carefully feel along the chest wall, up and over the collarbone, along the mastectomy scar, and in the underarm for any thickened areas or lumps. Look in the mirror for any signs of redness, swelling, or a rash near your scar. Become familiar with the landscape of your new breast. Recognize its irregularities after surgery, so you can distinguish them from any future changes that may occur.

Inform your oncologist or primary care physician of any of the following changes:

- sudden weight loss
- persistent abdominal pain
- chronic bone pain or tenderness
- chest pain or shortness of breath
- a rash, redness, or swelling that doesn't go away
- a change in overall health that lasts more than a couple of weeks

Monitor the opposite breast. If you've had breast cancer in one breast, you're at increased risk—about 1 percent each year—for developing cancer on the other side, so it's especially important to continue getting annual mammograms of your healthy breast. (If your natural breast is augmented, your mammogram should be performed by a technician who is trained to take images of implanted breasts.)

PART FOUR ○ FINDING ANSWERS, MAKING DECISIONS

CHAPTER SEVENTEEN

Searching for Dr. Right

If you can't hug your doctor, you've got the wrong one.

—**KAY, RECONSTRUCTION PATIENT**

You have a primary care physician who oversees your health, a team of medical professionals who coordinate your treatment, and specialists when you need them. When it comes to reconstruction, however, your plastic surgeon takes center stage. You can select your own doctors; that's your right. It's also a responsibility that requires effort on your part. Your choice of plastic surgeons is limited only by the restrictions of your health plan and your willingness to seek out Dr. Right.

Any competent surgeon can remove a breast. Rebuilding one isn't as easy. It takes skill and experience to tailor reconstruction to each woman's unique needs. Choosing an appropriate procedure is important—selecting the right plastic surgeon is even more critical to your outcome. A good surgeon is an artist and a sculptor; your post-mastectomy chest is his canvas and clay. Your new breasts are, quite literally, in his hands. He does the work, but you live with it. Some surgeons are good technicians, some are good artists. You want one who is both.

Shopping for a Surgeon

"Buyer beware" is sound advice when considering the services of any professional, including plastic surgeons. They're humans like the rest of us, and being human, they have different personalities, skills, and opinions. You probably wouldn't choose the first lawyer, financial advisor, or realtor you interviewed. It's the same with surgeons. Choosing a doctor is one of the most difficult personal decisions we make, yet studies show we actually spend more time choosing a car. You might randomly select a surgeon from the telephone directory or Internet and feel relieved to let him make all the decisions about which procedure you should have and what size your breasts should be. That's an easy decision, though it's one you might later regret. If you make the decision to pursue reconstruction, it makes sense to find the most experienced surgeon you can; someone who instills confidence and makes you feel comfortable, and whose work you admire.

When choosing a plastic surgeon, it's important to know what he's capable of giving you. Surgeons usually perform only certain procedures; very few are qualified in all methods of reconstruction. When a surgeon downplays one technique or the other, it may be because he feels it's not in your best interest, or because he isn't experienced doing it. If the first surgeon you see does only implant reconstruction with tissue expanders, he may not mention that direct-to-implant is also an option or that you have enough abdominal fat to rebuild your breasts. In your search for someone who is experienced with DIEP flap reconstruction, you might find surgeons who offer only TRAM or latissimus dorsi procedures, which are more common. Even if you eventually choose the surgeon you consulted with first, it's worth the time and effort to make sure he's the one for you. It's a bit like hunting for the right pair of shoes: there's a big selection and not every one will be a good fit. If at first you don't succeed, keep shopping.

> *The mastectomy surgeon recommended a plastic surgeon, and that's who I saw. I never thought of looking for other surgeons. He told me how he would rebuild my breasts and I agreed. Months later, I spoke to another woman who had reconstruction with an entirely different technique that sounded much better. Why didn't my surgeon mention that one?* —Lanie

Five Characteristics of an Ideal Plastic Surgeon

As you consult with different surgeons, look for five important characteristics.

1. *Skill.* There's no such thing as a typical reconstruction, because each woman is different. It takes skill and experience to rebuild and fine-tune a breast to get the very best result. Never judge a surgeon's skill by

her brochure or website. Depend on her qualifications, feedback from other patients, photos of her work, and your own confidence in the information she provides.

2. *Compassion.* You're more than a statistic on a chart, and you deserve to be treated respectfully and as an individual. A good surgeon cares about your expectations. He willingly repeats or clarifies information, is sympathetic to your concerns, and reacts to your anxiety with compassion. Ideally, you want someone who is proficient with both the technical and the non-technical aspects of care—not one or the other.

3. *Communication.* "My doctor doesn't listen to me" is a frequent complaint in patient satisfaction surveys. Your surgeon should talk with you, not to you, and give you his undivided attention. He ought to care and pay attention to what you want, rather than dictating how he intends to handle your reconstruction. He should explain terms and procedures so that you can understand them, and should patiently answer your questions even when you ask him to repeat something.

4. *Rapport.* It's important to find a surgeon you like. You'll have many questions and concerns throughout the process, and you need to feel comfortable voicing them. One surgeon may be too aggressive, another too impersonal for your taste. Your surgeon should never be condescending, abrupt, or rude.

5. *Honesty.* Look for someone who describes what you can realistically expect, rather than what she thinks you want to hear. If you have your heart set on D-cup implants, she should tell you whether your skin can be expanded sufficiently to accommodate that size. Leaning toward a tissue flap? Your surgeon ought to candidly describe what you can expect from the operation and recovery and how you'll look afterward. Think twice if a surgeon promises "You'll be as good as new" or "Your breasts will be perfect." You should be honest, too. Say what's on your mind, rather than what you think she expects.

My surgeon put me at ease by patiently answering all my questions. He smiled a lot, spoke slowly, and explained several different ways the reconstruction might be done. I felt I was talking to a trusted friend. —Cameran

I was so put off by my surgeon, I skipped my last appointment. He seemed more interested in me as his "creation" than as a person with cancer. He refused to accept that I didn't want big breasts. 　　　　*—Alicia*

I saw three different surgeons, who recommended three different techniques! One wanted to reconstruct my breast with implants, another wanted to use tissue from my back, and the third said I would have better results using my abdominal fat. 　　　　*—Betty*

Your Pre-appointment Footwork

Where do you find Dr. Right? Hospitals and universities with medical centers often have departments devoted specifically to breast cancer surgery, and many have excellent reconstruction staff. Hospital and recovery room nurses are great sources of information and often have firsthand experience with surgeons' work. Personal feedback is always preferable to an "eeney meeney miney moe" selection method. It's always nice to have a report from someone who's already been through reconstruction, preferably involving the same technique you're considering. Ask other women which surgeons they do or don't recommend and why. Reach to Recovery will put you in touch with women in your area who'll share their insights into the reconstruction experience and give you feedback about their plastic surgeons (call your local ACS office for information about the program). Or hop online to the American Society of Plastic Surgeons (www.plasticsurgery.org), the largest professional organization of reconstructive surgeons, to search by zip code or name. Check this book's companion website (www.breastrecon .com) for surgeons who offer direct-to-implant or microsurgical reconstruction. Make a list of reconstructive surgeons, then consult with at least two or three before selecting your Dr. Right. If possible, choose one who specializes in breast reconstruction—you don't want your new breasts to be made by a cosmetic surgeon who primarily provides facelifts, mommy makeovers, or other cosmetic procedures and seldom performs breast reconstruction.

Before you schedule an appointment. Now do some initial research for each of the surgeons on your list. First, check their websites or call their offices to ask a few key questions.

- Is the doctor accepting new patients?
- Does the doctor accept your insurance?
- What breast reconstruction procedures does he perform?
- How much experience does he have with each procedure?
- Does he work with a breast surgeon who is experienced with nipple-sparing mastectomy (if that is what you'd like)?
- What is his hospital affiliation?

Verify certification. Believe it or not, physicians don't need to be certified to perform plastic surgery. In most states—here's a frightening thought—any licensed physician can perform plastic surgery. While certification doesn't guarantee proficiency, it's a good starting place. To be certified by the ASPS, for example, a surgeon must graduate from an accredited medical school, complete a five-year residency of general and plastic surgery, practice for at least two years, and successfully complete oral and written exams. Verify certification for the surgeons you are considering at the American Board of Medical Specialties (www.abms.org).

Schedule a consultation. After weeding out individuals who don't take your insurance, don't provide the procedure you want, or can be ruled out for various other reasons, you're ready to arrange consultations with the top three or four surgeons on your list. (Scheduling an appointment early in the day, if that works for you, will give you a better chance of seeing the doctor on time.) Ask the receptionist how much time you'll have with the surgeon—if your consultation will be less than 30 minutes, ask for a longer appointment. The time will fly by as the surgeon examines you and describes various reconstructive procedures. Good plastic surgeons keep busy. If your mastectomy date is quickly approaching, let the receptionist know; she may be able to fit you in. In the meantime, interview other surgeons on your list.

Making the Most of Your Consultation

Your consultation appointment will usually begin with a review of your cancer diagnosis or treatment, genetic status (if you're pursuing preventive mastectomy), and overall medical history. The surgeon will check the quality and amount of your breast skin, and if you're considering flap reconstruction, she'll determine whether you have sufficient tissue at the donor site. The appointment should include a discussion of the reconstructive procedures the surgeon performs and what she thinks would work well for you (and why), based on your reconstructive preferences. You should also see her portfolio of before-and-after patient photos; this will probably reflect only her best work, so ask to see photos of not-so-good reconstructions as well, to get a broader perspective—not all surgeons are comfortable showing these or may not have them handy, but it doesn't hurt to ask. Use the following tips to make the most of your limited appointment time.

Come prepared. Even the best doctor can't explain all the nuances of a procedure or recovery in a single appointment. Learn as much as you can on your own, then make a list of the questions you would most like to have answered during the consultation. Ask the following questions to assess and compare the different ways surgeons approach reconstruction.

- Which reconstruction option is best for me and why?
- How many reconstructive surgeries of this type have you performed?
- How many do you do in a year?
- How many surgeries and office visits will be required, over what period of time?
- What are the possible side effects and risks from the procedure?
- Can my nipple and areola be preserved?
- Do you recommend surgery for my opposite breast for symmetry (if you're having unilateral reconstruction)?
- How many scars will I have and where will they be?
- What's the best result I can expect?
- How long will the surgery take and how long will I stay in the hospital?
- What will my recovery be like and how long will it take before I'm able to return to my normal routine?
- May I see your before-and-after patient photos with this procedure?
- May I speak with a couple of your patients who've had the same procedure you're recommending for me?
- What if I'm unhappy with my results?

- How much will my out-of-pocket costs be? (You may need to talk to the office billing manager about this.)

Bring your medical records. When you schedule an appointment, ask whether you should bring your pathology reports, mammograms, genetic test results, or other medical records for review. Then contact your doctor's office, hospital, or other facility to gather up everything you need.

Disclose medications, supplements, vitamins, and herbs. Your surgeon will advise which, if any, products you should discontinue and when you can resume taking them. This is very important, because some may interfere with circulation or healing. Include all prescribed and over-the-counter items. If you have several items to disclose, it's easier to hand your surgeon a list (table 17.1).

Don't be afraid to communicate The most successful consultation is interactive. Describe what you want from reconstruction and voice your concerns. If you would like smaller, larger, or rounder breasts, now is the time to say so. Don't be afraid to speak up if you need something explained, spelled, or repeated. Ask your surgeon to draw you a picture to clarify a procedure. Inquire about anything that concerns or confuses you, no matter how silly or insignificant it may seem.

Take notes. Experts say we forget 50 percent of what we hear in a doctor's office. That's not surprising, especially with a reconstruction consultation.

TABLE 17.1. Sample list of medications, supplements, vitamins, and herbs to report to your doctor before surgery

Medication	Dose	Frequency	Reason
Premarin	0.625 mg	Daily	Replace hormones
Simvastatin	20 mg	Daily	Manage cholesterol
Fish oil	1,200 mg	Daily	Manage cholesterol
Black cohosh	370 mg	Daily	Reduce hot flashes
Multivitamin	—	Daily	Aid nutritional health

The information and new terms can be overwhelming, especially when you're still dealing with treatment issues and trying to get used to the idea of mastectomy. Jot down or record the key points of your discussion so you can review them later. Better yet, bring someone with you. Four ears are better than two—your appointment buddy can take notes while you focus on listening. If you go to your appointment alone, use a tape recorder to capture your conversation with the surgeon.

Let it all sink in. Never feel pressured to make a decision about a surgeon or to schedule an operation before you leave the office. Take time to let everything sink in and to think about what you've heard. Discuss your options with your partner or an impartial trusted friend to get another perspective.

The Value of a Second (or Third) Opinion

Reconstruction recommendations vary widely, depending on the plastic surgeon's area of expertise and preference. You have nothing to lose and everything to gain by getting a second, if not a third, opinion. (Most health care insurance will pay for a second opinion.) Contact your health insurance company to determine under what conditions additional consultation appointments are covered. Waiting for another opinion shouldn't offend a surgeon; it's standard practice with any major operation.

Another opinion is always a good idea, and it can be especially helpful if you're unsure or confused about how to proceed or if you want to consider another surgeon's approach and recommendation. You may end up choosing the first surgeon you speak with, but it's good to consider other ideas. Some women feel that female surgeons are more sympathetic and can relate to reconstruction issues better than men can. Women who are happy with their male plastic surgeons might disagree. It's best to evaluate each surgeon on his or her own merits—you be the judge of what's best for you. Remember, you're doing the hiring. You needn't feel compelled or coerced to have one surgeon or the other do your surgery, no matter how persuasive they are. If you're uncomfortable with a surgeon for any reason, find someone else. Keep looking until you're satisfied you've found your Dr. Right.

After much research and window shopping with each and every consultation, I found a plastic surgeon who was the perfect match for me in every sense. I was immediately struck by his casual demeanor and appreciated his reassurances, availability, track record, and references, yet it was his striking confidence that won me over. We reviewed many of his before-and-after pictures to gain a real sense of what I wanted. We discussed the expander method at great lengths and mutually felt this route would provide optimal reconstruction for me. He was there for all of my medical needs and always returned my phone calls and e-mails promptly. Most of all, he was an absolute perfectionist and I appreciated his artistic abilities. —Marie*

Tips for Travelers

You're lucky if you live in or close to a city with a great reconstructive surgeon. But the best reconstructive opportunity isn't always possible locally, particularly if you live in a small town or rural area. If the surgeons and techniques you want aren't available nearby, you'll need to decide whether you want to settle for the local expertise or travel for your reconstruction. Even though journeying to another city for your surgery involves more time, effort, and cost—your insurance won't pay for travel and hotel costs, and your out-of-pocket expense may be higher—if you are able to do so, you may consider it worthwhile to pack up for a few days to get the surgeon and procedure you want. Many reconstructive surgery practices, especially those that offer breast reconstruction exclusively, have patient relations coordinators who can facilitate consultation appointments, coordinate insurance coverage, and recommend hotels with which they've negotiated patient discounts. They'll also recommend a breast surgeon in the same city, so you won't need to search for someone to do your mastectomy. If you can manage it, you can drive or fly in for a consultation and return home the same day. If that doesn't work, you can swap information, including photos of your breasts and donor site, by e-mail, followed by a phone consultation. If you like what you hear, you can arrange an in-person consultation or schedule your surgery. Once your surgery date is on the calendar, you can complete all the necessary pre-op testing in your hometown, with a copy of the results forwarded to your distant plastic surgeon.

The surgeon's office will advise you of all the necessary travel require-ments. Generally, you'll need to be away from home for about a week: you'll have a pre-op appointment on the day before your surgery, then spend an overnight in the hospital for implant surgery or three to five days after flap surgery. After you're discharged, you'll need to remain in town (with fam-ily or friends or in a hotel) until your post-op appointment or until your surgeon clears you to return home. This time period varies, depending on the procedure you have and how well you recover. If you'll be flying home after a flap reconstruction, it's helpful to arrange for a wheelchair at the airport. You'll avoid long walks through the terminal and jostling crowds, and you'll be able to pre-board the airplane. Your surgeon should provide a letter stating you've had major surgery, just in case there are any questions about your drains as you go through security.

It may be hard to fathom traveling far from home to have surgery and all that this entails, but most women who do so don't require follow-up care once they return home. As a precaution, you should contact a local plastic surgeon or surgical oncologist before your reconstruction to ask whether they'll provide follow-up care if you need it.

CHAPTER EIGHTEEN

Paying for Your Reconstruction

Life isn't about waiting for the storm to pass, it's about learning to dance in the rain. —ANONYMOUS

If you've had a smooth relationship with your insurance company while dealing with breast cancer or other serious health issues, you're among the fortunate. Paying for your reconstruction is often not straightforward, even when you have insurance coverage. While numerous women have absolutely no problems at all with reconstruction-related insurance coverage, too many say that dealing with their insurers is almost as nerve-wracking as coping with a breast cancer diagnosis or the surgery itself.

In 1998, Congress passed the Women's Health and Cancer Rights Act, requiring group health plans that pay for mastectomy to also cover prostheses and reconstructive procedures (table 18.1). Also known as Janet's Law, the WHCRA is named after Janet Franquet, a woman who was denied reconstructive surgery after mastectomy because her insurance company considered it to be cosmetic rather than medically necessary. Her surgeon generously performed her surgery for free. Franquet pursued a lengthy appeals process, which she eventually won.

The WHCRA recognizes breast reconstruction as more than cosmetic surgery, but it stops short of guaranteeing your absolute choice in the matter. Although the law doesn't extend to Medicare and Medicaid, both programs also cover reconstructive surgery. To learn more about the law, search for "WHCRA" at the Department of Labor's Employee Benefits Security Administration website (www.askebsa.dol.gov). Your state's health insurance agency or insurance commissioner can provide details of additional laws concerning mastectomy and reconstruction where you live.

The Affordable Care Act of 2010 prohibits health insurers from imposing lifetime dollar limits on essential benefits, such as hospital stays. The law also restricts and phases out the annual cap that a health plan can place

TABLE 18.1. Requirements and limits of the Women's Health and Cancer Rights Act (1998)

Requires insurers to cover:	Does *not*:
Breast prostheses and special mastectomy bras	Require insurance companies to pay for mastectomy
All stages of breast reconstruction*	Set payment rates, or guarantee specific procedures or choice of surgeons
Additional procedures to achieve symmetry, including modification of the healthy breast after unilateral reconstruction	Apply to all plans; certain government and church plans are exempt (some cover mastectomy and reconstruction anyway)
Treatment for complications from mastectomy or reconstruction	Provide retroactive coverage; if you weren't insured with your current plan before January 1999 or you had your mastectomy before that time, your current insurer isn't obligated to cover your reconstruction now

*If you change insurance companies and your new plan covers mastectomy, it must also cover reconstruction.

on most of your benefits, including breast reconstruction, and eliminates these limits entirely from 2014 onward. (Some policies and plans that were issued on or before March 23, 2010, are grandfathered and don't have to comply with some provisions of the law.)

Are You Covered?

Dealing proactively with your insurance company before your surgery is a smart move that most likely will avoid unpleasant payment surprises. Never assume your health insurance will automatically cover your reconstruction. Check your benefits handbook, plan document, or policy to determine what is covered and what isn't. Call the customer service department if you need further clarification. Your most valuable ally is the insurance specialist in your plastic surgeon's office. While the insurance experience may be new to you, she deals with preauthorizations, payments, denials, and related issues every day, and has probably already had experience dealing with your insurance company. She'll help you navigate the insurance maze and may do much of the footwork to arrange payment with your insurer.

Questions for your health insurance company:

- Does my plan cover mastectomy? (If the answer is yes, it must also cover reconstruction.)
- How many "second" opinions are covered?
- How should I obtain preauthorization for my surgery?
- Am I limited to in-network surgeons and services?
- If I travel to another surgeon who specializes in a particular technique not available within my network, what expenses will be covered?
- What are my total out-of-pocket costs if I go to an out-of-network surgeon?
- Is there a limit to the amount of coverage provided?
- Is my hospital stay covered? If so, for how many days?
- Are the other providers involved in my surgery covered?
- Will all bills be paid directly to providers?

How much will you have to pay? Without a standard fee structure, costs for mastectomy and reconstruction vary widely, depending on where your surgeon practices and the procedure you choose: the cost of an implant or DIEP reconstruction in New York may be quite different from the cost for the same procedure in San Diego or Des Moines. A plastic surgeon might charge $5,000 for implant reconstruction and $100,000 or more for a microsurgical flap—and that doesn't include costs for the anesthesiologist, pathologist, operating room, and hospital stay.

Like all businesses, health care insurers limit services to control costs and increase profits. They pay according to their own fee schedule, which is generally only a fraction of a surgeon's "sticker price." In some cases, health carriers reimburse surgeons at the same or similar rates regardless of the reconstructive procedures they perform. Insurance reimbursements for flap procedures are woefully inadequate, considering the time and effort involved; typically, it's not much more than what is paid for an implant reconstruction. (Coincidentally, implant reconstruction has a higher reoperation rate and, in the long term, may cost more.) This is bad news for patients, because poor reimbursement rates encourage surgeons to discontinue flap reconstruction in favor of implant procedures (augmentation or reconstruction) or other cosmetic surgery, or to simply stop accepting health insurance altogether. A survey of U.S. plastic surgeons found that although 90 percent considered breast reconstruction to be personally rewarding and nearly all enjoyed the technical aspects of the procedures, 43 percent limited the number of breast reconstructions they performed, because of poor reimbursement.[1]

Working within your health plan. If your health plan covers mastectomy and reconstruction, it must do so under its overall guidelines. You still have to pay any *deductibles* and *co-payments* routinely required for office visits or other surgeries. In other words, if your plan normally pays 80 percent of medical services and you pay the remaining 20 percent, the same schedule applies to your reconstructive expenses. Be sure to follow your plan's process for requesting reconstruction, including preauthorization.

Choosing an *in-network* surgeon is to your financial advantage and will limit your *out-of-pocket costs* to whatever deductible and co-pay you are ordinarily responsible for. In-network providers agree to accept predetermined fees for services they provide; this is usually much less than their customary fees, and they write off the remaining unpaid balance. Your plan may limit your choice of surgeons to those who practice locally, or it may include surgeons in other states.

Out-of-network providers don't have payment agreements with the insurer and aren't as likely to write off a balance due. That translates into higher out-of-pocket costs for you. A surgeon may accept a combination of your insurer's offered payment and your co-pay as payment in full. If he does not, you may be responsible for "balance billing" to make up the difference. It's important to determine your total out-of-pocket expenses before you schedule surgery. If your surgeon doesn't accept insurance and advises you to pay him in advance and then seek reimbursement from your health insurer, realize your financial risk: your insurance company may compensate you for only a small part of the amount you paid, or none at all.

You may deduct a percentage of your out-of-pocket medical expenses from your state and federal income taxes, including costs related to your breast cancer treatment and reconstruction, and all other health-related expenses you pay during the tax year. Check with your tax professional or see IRS Publication 502 for a complete list of deductible expenses.

Appealing When the Answer Is No

Several days after your preauthorization request, a letter arrives from your insurance company. You're expecting an approval, but find a refusal instead: your request has been denied. Angry, frustrated, and feeling helpless, women often give up at this point. Is it worth the effort to challenge your insurance company's decision? Yes! You have nothing to lose and so much to gain. Despite federal and state laws protecting a woman's right to breast reconstruction, denials occur more frequently than you might imagine. If you feel strongly about overturning your denial, you must act as your own advocate. You should know before you begin that attempting to get your insurer to recant can be frustrating and time consuming. But health care organizations aren't perfect; nor are they invincible. Other women have won appeals and you may be able to do the same, depending on the circumstances—almost half of all health claim denials are overturned when they are appealed. And here's a little secret: sometimes simply appealing the decision gets it overturned. If the company realizes it's made a mistake or feels it's more cost effective to grant your request than fight it, you'll win.

Your health insurance company must state the reason for refusal in its notification to you. It may be difficult to find rhyme or reason for the logic behind the decision, but all health insurance policies are different and coverage varies, depending on many variables. You're least likely to encounter problems when you choose an in-network surgeon who provides traditional implant, lat flap, or TRAM flap reconstruction. Requests for newer implant and flap procedures and out-of-network services are more likely to be refused. Here's how to go about appealing a denial.

Follow the process. Challenging a denial is your legal right. If you're going to appeal, you must follow exactly your plan's appeal procedure as it is described in your denial letter and your benefits manual. The process will involve internal appeals handled by your insurance company. By law, employer-provided insurance plans may have no more than two appeal levels. At the first level, appeals are typically decided by a claims reviewer and signed off by a medical professional; a denial is least likely to be over-turned at this level. The second appeal is considered by a review panel that includes at least one physician in the same specialty you requested—in this case, plastic surgery. If your insurance carrier allows it, try an in-person appeal at this level, which can be more effective than a written appeal. Sub-mit all paperwork on time to meet the deadlines for each level of appeal—if your policy states you have 30 days to appeal a decision, you're not likely to be granted an extension. Send your appeal by certified mail to the appro-priate contact listed in your denial letter.

Focus on the reason for denial. Call your insurance company and request a copy of the medical opinion on which your denial is based; this should be the focus of your request for reconsideration. Also, request a case manager for your appeal. She'll become familiar with your case, and contacting her directly will save you the time and hassle of having to go through customer service representatives each time you call. In most cases, your denial will be based on one of the following reasons:

- "Benefit not provided" means your plan doesn't provide the service you requested. Check your benefits summary to see whether mastectomy is a covered benefit. If it is, the insurer must also provide coverage for recon-struction. Include a copy of the WHCRA with your appeal letter, stating that the denial appears to be in violation of the law.
- "Not medically necessary" means that the insurer doesn't consider your reconstructive procedure to be necessary for your continued good health. If your insurer vetoes your request for prophylactic mastectomy, for example, ask your oncologist, primary care physician, or medical geneticist (or all three) to write letters describing your family history of breast cancer and confirming your high-risk status. Attach studies show-ing that prophylactic bilateral mastectomy is an effective and accepted risk management protocol for high-risk women.
- "Out-of-network" is one of the most common reasons for rejecting a

reconstruction request and one of the most difficult appeals to win, especially if the procedure you want is provided by an in-network surgeon. Unless you can show that your request is medically necessary, you're not likely to have a denial for out-of-network benefits reversed. Your insurer will most likely refuse your request to go to an out-of-network surgeon across the country for your GAP reconstruction, for instance, if an in-network surgeon also provides the same procedure. However, if GAP is the only procedure for which you're a candidate (perhaps your implants failed after radiation and you're too thin for any other flap reconstruction) and no in-network surgeons perform GAP, you have a very good argument. If you can obtain a letter or an e-mail from an in-network surgeon validating your decision, so much the better. The same approach applies to DIEP, hip flaps, direct-to-implant procedures, and other types of breast reconstruction.

- "Procedure is experimental" means your carrier doesn't recognize or accept the procedure you requested. The company may be unfamiliar with a particular type of reconstruction, and once educated, might reverse its denial. This may be the case if you prefer DIEP, GAP, TUG, direct-to-implant, or other newer reconstructive procedures that your carrier considers to be above and beyond the more traditional tissue expansion, lat flaps, and TRAM. Support your case with peer-reviewed studies and articles in medical journals that prove your requested procedure is established, bona fide, and safe. If your insurance carrier turns down your request for a DIEP reconstruction because in-network surgeons already provide TRAM procedures, point out the shorter hospital stay and fewer postoperative complications with DIEP. Cite Johns Hopkins Hospital, one of the most respected medical cancer facilities in the world, which no longer offers pedicled TRAM surgeries because DIEP is far superior. (Search for "reconstructive breast surgery options" at www.hopkinsmedicine.org for supporting documentation to include in your appeal.) One other circumstance may work in your favor: if you can show that other insurers in your area cover the procedure you want (your surgeon's billing coordinator can help with this), you may sway the company to change its opinion and, in doing so, help yourself and pave the way for other women who request the procedure in the future.

Unfortunately my insurance company is really dragging its corporate feet and has not yet authorized my PBM. Their "BRCA expert" seems very ill-informed so I am trying to look at this as an educational opportunity for them. If I cannot prevail, I will change to a new insurer in January.   —Samantha

Build your case. The hardest part of an appeal is crafting your response without letting your frustration and emotions get in the way. Although your reconstruction is a very personal matter for you, it's a business decision for your insurance company. And while it is disheartening to have your request refused, this is the time for logic to prevail. Resist the temptation to sit down and fire off an immediate angry response. Be aggressively persistent without being hostile. You have a better chance of succeeding if your appeal is brief and clear and includes fact-based evidence that clearly justifies your argument. Don't waste your time reiterating what the insurer already knows. Stick to the issue at hand, focusing on evidence that refutes the reason for rejection. Your plastic surgeon's office may provide sample letters that have worked successfully for other patients.

Start working on your appeal strategy soon after you receive notification of denial. Gather up all the information you need: applicable medical records, supporting letters from physicians, and research materials that help make your case. Top it off with a formal cover letter that includes:

- your insurance policy number
- your appeal claim number
- acknowledgment that you've received the denial
- a request for a "physician review," which means your appeal will be reviewed by a plastic surgeon
- a request for reconsideration

It doesn't hurt to ask your case manager to arrange a call between your plastic surgeon and the medical director who will be reviewing your appeal. (When surgeons actually speak together, a denial may be overturned.) Send copies of the entire package to your physician and your lawyer, if you have one, and to your government representatives (the latter probably won't help, but it can't hurt). Show a Cc to them in your cover letter to your insurer.

Ask for help. Don't be shy about asking your physicians to provide supportive letters or point you in the right direction for peer-reviewed studies and medical reports on the procedure you want. You can also search PubMed.gov, the U.S. National Library of Medicine's online repository of medical studies. The non-profit Patient Advocate Foundation (www .patientadvocate.org) will help you along the way, at no charge, and act as a liaison between you and your insurance company—the organization's website also has sample appeal letters.

Keep a paper trail. Keep copies of all written correspondence and a call log of your conversations with insurance company employees, noting the date, time, details of the discussion, and name of the employee. If a discrepancy comes up, you'll have supportive documentation.

When All Else Fails

In most states, once you've exhausted your insurer's appeals process (but not before), you can request an appeal with an external reviewer at the state level. This secondary appeal is conducted by an independent medical review board of plastic surgeons who are empowered to sustain or overrule an insurance company's decision—the insurer's denial will probably be upheld if the panel finds it conforms to state law and abides by the company's stated rules of coverage. The verdict may take 30 to 60 days; you can request an expedited decision if you show sufficient cause for an emergency ruling.

Fully insured plans (in which your employer buys health coverage from an insurance company) are regulated by state laws, so any external appeal process is administered by the state. Your appeal rights may vary, depending on the type of health insurance plan you have and the process required by the state in which you live. Self-insured plans (your employer pays claims from its own resources, even if it contracts with an insurance company to administer the plan) are governed by the Employee Retirement Income Security Act (ERISA), a federal law; these plans aren't required to comply with all state laws. Therefore, if your plan is self-insured, you may have no appeal rights at the state level. You can learn more about state and federal insurance laws and find information about appeals online at the Cancer Legal Resource Center (www.cancerlegalresourcecenter.org) and the U.S. Department of Health and Human Services (www.healthcare.gov). Check with your state's department of insurance to learn more about the appeal process. Find contact information for your state at the National Insurance Commission's website (www.naic.org/state_web_map.htm).

The Affordable Care Act of 2010 mandates impartial internal and external appeal processes for everyone who is covered by a plan that was created after March 23, 2010. States must provide independent and impartial reviewers who meet certain standards, keep written records, and aren't affected by conflicts of interest. If you're not protected by a state law, you can appeal to a federal external review program. If the external reviewer agrees with your appeal, your health care plan must pay for the benefit in question. If your insurance company's denial is upheld, your only other option is to pursue legal action. It may be worth the money to pay for an hour's consultation with a health insurance lawyer to determine her applicable fees, success with similar appeals, and whether she thinks you have a case. If you can't afford the fee, contact your state bar association to inquire about lawyers who will write an appeal letter for you at no charge. You may also contact your state legislator or insurance commissioner, if you feel you're being treated unfairly or illegally.

Help for the uninsured. Reconstruction can be expensive, and for most women, it's probably cost prohibitive without insurance or financial assistance. If you don't have health insurance and you can't afford mastectomy and reconstruction, you may be eligible for programs for low-income and uninsured women. Contact your local medical center, teaching facility, or ACS branch office to see whether they're aware of special local funding programs or know of plastic surgeons who donate reconstructive services for a few women each year (many surgeons do). My Hope Chest (www .myhopechest.org), the United Breast Cancer Foundation (www.ubcf .info), and other charitable breast cancer organizations may offer financial help for your surgery. If paying out of pocket is your only alternative, many surgeons offer reduced fees and payment schedules for breast cancer survivors. CareCredit (www.carecredit.com) offers payment plans for medical services, including breast reconstruction, for as long as 60 months.

My insurance company was great. My benefits manual outlined how
mastectomy and reconstruction were covered. My in-network surgeons

performed the procedure I wanted and I didn't give it a second thought. I never even saw a bill, so I assume everything was paid. —Dawn

I was told by my insurance company's customer service department that PBM wasn't covered under any circumstances. I was so angry, I stomped into my boss's office and told her I thought it was incredibly unfair. She contacted our Human Resources director, who arranged a call for me with a manager at the insurance company. When I explained my BRCA status, the manager said that sometimes the customer service personnel made mistakes, and assured me that my PBM would be covered. It was a good thing I pursued this, because my PBM and reconstruction were both paid for without problems. —Judy

After seeing my friend's fabulous reconstruction results, I was determined to go to her plastic surgeon, who happened to be in another state and was out-of-network for me, but my health insurance company denied my request. Even though I spent hours talking with people at the insurance company and writing appeals, I couldn't get them to change their minds. —Trish

Other Types of Insurance

If you're employed by a company with 50 or more employees, the Family Medical Leave Act (www.dol.gov, search for "FMLA") entitles you to at least 12 weeks of unpaid medical leave. (You can also break up the 12 weeks into smaller increments, such as taking off every other Friday to recover from your expander fills.) You must have worked for your employer for at least 1,250 hours in the previous 12 months. If you take FMLA leave, your employer must provide full health benefits while you're away from the job and restore you to your previous position or a similar job with the same salary and benefits when you return.

If you have a short-term disability plan before your surgery, it will work like an insurance plan for your wages: depending on the amount of your premium and the terms of your policy, the policy pays you a portion or all of your regular work pay while you're unable to return to work.

CHAPTER NINETEEN

Making Difficult Decisions

We either make ourselves miserable or we make ourselves strong. The amount of work is the same.

—CARLOS CASTANEDA

You may have a team of family, friends, soul sisters, and medical professionals supporting your pending mastectomy and reconstruction, but guess who most influences your decisions?

You do.

Reconstruction can be an exciting and terrifying possibility. The decisions you face are complicated and intensely personal, and no one can make them for you. With mastectomy looming ahead, you may know precisely how you want to proceed. More likely, you're living in a state of uncertainty about what to do and when to do it. Should you have reconstruction? Is nipple-sparing mastectomy an option for you? Would implants or a tissue flap give you a better result? Should you travel for a procedure you can't have locally or for a more experienced surgeon who can offer you a better possibility than a hometown surgeon? Making your own informed decisions about reconstruction can help restore the lack of control you may feel during your diagnosis and treatment. So how do you find answers when you're not even sure of the right questions?

Ten Steps in the Right Direction

Making the best personal decisions may seem like a tall order, considering the many procedures and options you need to learn about and sort through. With so much to absorb, you may feel you're stuck on a merry-go-round of endless terms and concepts. The following tips will help you make your way through the onslaught of information and what-ifs in front of you.

1. *Establish a positive attitude.* Consider your research an empowering action rather than an awful chore. Your investigative efforts will help you make a confident decision.

2. *Take time to learn.* When it comes to surgery, informed is always better than impetuous. Being informed about the benefits and limitations of various reconstructive options gives you something special: the power of choice. Breast cancer isn't a medical emergency for most women, and you needn't make a decision that you haven't had time to consider thoroughly. Unless you've been diagnosed with an aggressive breast cancer, taking two to three weeks to learn about reconstruction probably won't adversely affect your health. You should, of course, discuss this research interval with your medical team. If you're having preventive mastectomy, you have the luxury of time to consider reconstruction. You would probably compare loan rates before financing a home, and get to know someone pretty well before marrying them or forming a business partnership—it's only logical to approach a decision concerning your physical and emotional well-being with the same scrutiny. To use a corny football analogy, don't sit on the bench. Suit up and get in the game. Be your own advocate.

3. *Recruit a study buddy.* Having a research helper saves time and provides a second perspective. Your spouse or partner may be the best person for the task; sharing the experience helps to build understanding, commitment, and compassion. If this isn't practical, ask a relative or close friend to assist you.

4. *Be patient and persistent.* Take things one step at a time. Don't let frustration get you down. When you think you can't absorb any more information (but need to), take a break. Have lunch with a friend, listen to your favorite music, see a movie, or go for a walk.

5. *Deal with data.* As much as possible, weed out the influences of media hype, personal anecdote, and urban myth. Make your decisions based on the facts of a particular procedure and surgeon's expertise.

6. *Know when to stop.* At some point, you need to assess all the data you've gathered and make your decision. If you're still unsure, it may be best to delay your reconstruction.

7. *Sort through your options.* When you first learn that mastectomy is a certainty, you may already have a particular reconstruction procedure

in mind. Even so, it's still wise to consider all the possibilities available to you. Understanding your options will demystify reconstruction, replacing the unknown with the expected and reducing your anxiety about the various ways your breasts can be rebuilt. Along the way, you may discover that reconstruction can give you better breasts than you expected, or you may find that it requires more than you're willing to go through.

8. *Take time to absorb.* Even after you make the decision to have reconstruction, you may still have doubts about the procedure. It's not unusual to feel this way. Experts say shock, denial, anger, and depression

TABLE 19.1. Fill-in table to assess your breast reconstruction options

Implants or flaps?	Procedure	Acceptable procedure?	Acceptable recovery?	Available locally?	Sufficient donor tissue?	Insurance coverage?
Implants	Expander-to-implant				_____	
	Hybrid expander				_____	
	Direct-to-implant				_____	
Tissue flaps	Latissimus dorsi (lat)					
	Attached TRAM					
	Free TRAM					
	Muscle-sparing TRAM					
	DIEP					
	SGAP					
	IGAP					
	TUG					
	Hip flap					

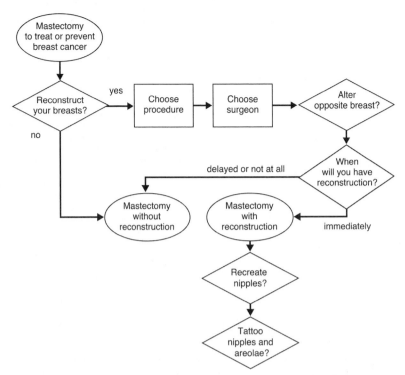

FIGURE 19.1. Considering breast reconstruction requires several key decisions.

typically come before acceptance. Meanwhile, life goes on: there's work to be done, a home to manage, perhaps kids to hug and pets to feed. Give yourself time to let everything sink in and reflect on what you've learned.

9. *Prioritize your alternatives.* Your choice of a particular reconstructive procedure will be influenced by many factors. Perhaps you don't want to have additional scars from a flap procedure, or you don't want to try implants after radiation. Your priority might be to have the quickest reconstruction possible or the best possible results . . . or both. Perhaps you're not compelled to replace your breasts at all. As you consider all the variables, use a process of elimination to whittle the possibilities down to procedures that interest you and for which you are a candidate (table 19.1).

10. *Make your decision.* Consider the input of loved ones, physicians, and other women who have had a mastectomy, then listen to your own instincts. Others may influence what you decide, but you're the one who must go through the surgery and recovery, and you're the one who will live with the results. It's you, after all, who best knows your body. With many options available, the tough decisions—the what, when, who, why, and how of breast reconstruction—are up to you (figure 19.1). Weigh

all of the pros and cons for each procedure to choose the one you feel is best. Whatever you decide is the right choice.

My mother was diagnosed with breast cancer at age 45 and died five years later when I was sixteen, so my high-risk status raised a host of monsters in my head. I was initially terrified and overwhelmed by the information, then decided quickly to have prophylactic oophorectomy and mastectomy—I did not want my two children to lose their mother as early as I did. I considered implant reconstruction, the only type available locally, but I was interested in flap reconstruction as soon as I learned about it. I was lucky to connect with someone who had already interviewed a number of the doctors in my state and nationally who do flap procedures, and to benefit from her extensive research. The more I learned about flap surgery, the more I knew it was the best choice for me. Using my own tissue for a more natural look and feel, and not having implants that would need to be replaced down the road, were the most important factors. Once I saw a friend's beautiful DIEP flap reconstruction, my fears about the surgery were greatly relieved. I know that combined with nipple-sparing mastectomy, it was the best balance of risk reduction and cosmetic result.—Sonya

I agonized over my reconstruction choice, but after thinking and rethinking my options, I ultimately chose implants, because I just couldn't accommodate the childcare and time away from work a flap surgery would require.
                                                              —Rachel

Other Sources of Information and Inspiration

Just a few years ago, reconstruction choices were limited and information was hard to come by. With a few clicks of your mouse, you can now bring an amazing assortment of information and personal experience directly to your desktop, if you know where to look for the bits and pieces. And it's all free. Medical reports, articles, and personal reconstruction journals await on the Internet. Before-and-after color photos of women who have had mastectomy and reconstruction can be found on websites of plastic surgeons and the American Society of Plastic Surgeons (www.plasticsur gery.org). Sorting through all this information can be overwhelming, however, and before you know it, you may have spent days in front of your computer but feel no closer to getting the answers you need. You'll save time by narrowing your search to specific terms. Searching for "breast reconstruction," for example, brings up 2,780,000 references (in 2005, the same search produced 29,000 references—just to show you how much more information is now available), while a more specific search for "direct-to-implant breast reconstruction" produces 41,000 listings. Always use credible information sources. Bookmark your favorite websites for easy return. If you're curious and have the fortitude, you can watch actual breast and nipple reconstruction operations at ORlive (www.orlive.com) and YouTube (www.youtube.com).

Mastectomy and reconstruction used to be topics women kept to themselves. While some still prefer to keep their experiences private, many are happy to share the details of their reconstruction and recovery online—look on message boards, in chat rooms, and on social sites such as Facebook and Twitter. Discussion groups at Susan G. Komen for the Cure (www.komen.org), Cancer Support Network (csn.cancer.org), and Johns Hopkins Medicine (www.hopkinsbreastcenter.org/services/ask _expert) frequently have postings related to reconstruction. The FORCE message boards (www.facingourrisk.org) are one of the most informative and supportive online neighborhoods, particularly concerning reconstruction. Members have been through every imaginable breast cancer and reconstruction experience. No matter where you are in the journey, there's a huge sisterhood of previvors and survivors with reconstruction experience who have "been there and done that" and are ready and willing to lend a virtual shoulder. Having experienced the same emotional roller coaster and confusion, they can relate to what you're feeling better than anyone else. One caveat about discussions of mastectomy and breast reconstruction on blogs and message boards: women are often passionate about their reconstruction, whether they're happy or dissatisfied with the results. Realize that someone else's experience won't necessarily be yours, and her choice may not be the best solution for you. Try not to substitute personal opinion for medical advice or use the experiences of just one or two women to make your decision.

Local support groups can also be helpful. Contact your nearest ACS office, hospital, or breast cancer center to see whether they sponsor reconstruction discussion groups, seminars, or lectures. Your library and bookstore shelves offer memoirs of women who have gone through the same emotional upheaval that you're experiencing, including four exceptional examples:

In the Family (DVD), by Joanna Rudnick, documents the 27-year-old film-maker's experiences and conflicts dealing with the impact of a positive BRCA gene test.

Pretty Is What Changes is an award-winning memoir by 34-year-old TV writer Jessica Queller and how she dealt with difficult decisions about her breasts when she tested positive for a BRCA mutation just 11 months after she lost her mother to ovarian cancer.

Spinning Straw into Gold, by psychotherapist and breast cancer survivor Ronnie Kaye, explains how to deal with the emotional side effects of breast cancer.

Why I Wore Lipstick to My Mastectomy, by Geralyn Lucas, chronicles a 27-year-old woman's unusual and inspiring approach to her mastectomy and reconstruction in our beauty-obsessed culture.

CHAPTER TWENTY

Information for Family and Friends

Trouble is a part of life, and if you don't share it, you don't give the person who loves you a chance to love you enough.

—DINAH SHORE

If someone you care about is facing breast reconstruction, your support will be a welcome gift. Surgery and recovery can be difficult roads to walk alone, and while you can't go through the experience for her, you can rally to her side, providing love and strength to see her through.

Hints for Family Members

For parents. It's difficult to see your daughter struggle with life-altering decisions, pain, and anxiety, especially if you've faced a similar situation yourself. You probably would be willing to trade places and spare her the experience, if you could. You can help in the weeks before surgery, which can be nerve-wracking for her. Join in as she researches mastectomy and reconstruction—read through this book so you'll know what to expect. Help her put her house in order before surgery, and arrange to get things done during her recovery. Most important of all, help by supporting whatever decisions she makes about mastectomy and reconstruction, even if you disagree. Understand that even though these surgeries aren't life-threatening, both require sacrifice and recovery.

For siblings. Now is the time to support your sister, whether you live down the street or across the country. It's not the best time to bring up family grudges or disagreements, but it's the perfect time to let your words or deeds show that you care. Call frequently to make her laugh when she's down. Buy her a pair of pretty pajamas (button in the front) or something that will comfort her in the hospital and when she returns home. Bring or send her a teddy bear, flowers, or a balloon bouquet. If she's a mom, shift your schedule to care for your nieces and nephews. Take them to school, the zoo, or the movies. Attend their sports activities when your sister cannot. Be supportive; stay in touch to express your good thoughts and encouragement.

Food for Thought for Partners and Spouses

Mastectomy and reconstruction are feared events that you know are possible and you hoped you'd never have to face. But now you do. Unless you've experienced a loved one's surgery and recovery, you may be overwhelmed and scared, and you may feel clueless about how you can best help her. This may be frustrating for you, particularly if your usual approach to problems is to try to fix them. You can't fix this situation—you can't change the fact that she needs a mastectomy and you can't shorten her recovery—you can do many things to help her as she goes through the experience.

Be her sounding board. An old saying goes, "God gave us two ears but only one mouth. Some people say that's because he wanted us to spend twice as much time listening as talking." Listening is a skill, and now, more than ever, your mate will appreciate your sympathetic ear. Give her your full attention as she expresses her concerns and asks your opinion about the many "ifs" involved in reconstruction decisions. Listen to her fears, issues, and questions with an open mind. Consider why she wants to travel to a distant city for reconstruction when there are plastic surgeons in your hometown, or why she's leaning in favor of tissue flap reconstruction when implants would be quicker. You don't have to—and shouldn't—make decisions for her, but it will be a comfort for her to share ideas with you and know she can confide in you.

Be her partner. You may not be able to rescue your partner, but you can join her on the journey and let her know you're there for her. Let her know that you'll go through this life-changing experience together, even if you're not quite sure how to help her. Be an extra set of ears at her doctor's appointments—ask questions, take notes, and look at before-and-after patient photos together. Then discuss what you've learned when you get home. Learn with her about reconstructive options and what to expect from recovery, so that you can approach these issues as a team. Search the Internet for helpful articles, then print them out so you can read and discuss them together. While she's recovering, arrange (and rearrange) pillows so she can rest comfortably. Maybe a gentle back rub would be just the ticket. Run interference with friends who call to see how she's doing, and make sure the kids don't jump up on Mommy. Learn how to empty her drains. Your attentiveness will be immensely reassuring. Comfort her if she needs to have a good cry or to just vent about what she's having to endure. Take time to read *Breast Cancer Husband* by Marc Silver, a revealing look into how a woman's surgery and recovery affects her partner, and tips for coping with the experience.

Be her communicator. Say yes when friends ask whether they can help. Coordinate a brigade to deliver meals, run errands, and arrange childcare. Send e-mail status reports to close family and friends, so you won't be inundated with calls to check on the patient. Take advantage of the Internet and social networking sites such as Facebook and Twitter to stay connected. Create a blog or use CaringBridge (www.caringbridge.com).

Be her cheerleader. Although most women recover from reconstruction without additional problems, the road to recovery is sometimes littered with setbacks. Initially, your partner may be fragile, fatigued, and anxious—impatient to have recovery over and done with. A small roadblock can seem enormous. Respect her feelings when she's disappointed because her drains need to remain a while longer. Understand when she's not upbeat because her expanders are uncomfortable or she's developed an infection. Listen to her concerns and let her know that although these things feel devastating now, they can be corrected and will get better. Reassure her if she's disappointed with how her new breast looks. Remind her to give reconstruction adequate time to improve, and support her if she wants to pursue corrective action. Let her talk when she feels like it, and respect her need for silence when she doesn't. Be there for her, whether she's angry, impatient, or scared. Hug her gently when she is overwhelmed or frustrated.

Be her lover. Some women have no problem at all with the transition back to a normal sex life after reconstruction, while others feel irreparably changed. Be patient if your partner's ordeal has left her nervous about intimacy; she may feel insecure about her breasts or how she looks. Use actions and words to reassure her that mastectomy and reconstruction are not the end of your sex life together. Tell her that you still desire her and still consider her whole—these are powerful, reassuring words at a time when she may question her own femininity.

Your partner needs to heal physically and emotionally. She may have trouble with one or the other, or both. Realize that while her new breast might feel the same to you, it won't be the same to her. Because she won't have the same sensation she's used to, in much of her reconstructed breast, including her nipples, she'll be unable to feel your touch—that may change some aspects of your intimacy. Encourage her to talk about how she feels, and approach troublesome issues together. Don't be afraid to include her breasts in your lovemaking; focus on the areas where she has the most feeling.

> *When my wife faced mastectomy, I felt a deep and strong conviction that all I wanted was for her to make choices that would most increase her chances of survival, and I would support the decisions she made. Although I knew that I loved her with or without breasts, I was glad that she decided to have reconstruction because I thought it would be important for her self image. When the reconstruction was new, I felt her grief when she had no sensation and said that it felt strange when I touched her breasts. I wanted to caress them because they were a part of her; however, I quickly learned to first stroke around and between her breasts where she had feeling before touching the area that lacked sensation. In this way, we were both able to appreciate a new intimacy that included her reconstructed chest. Now, thirteen years later, I rarely think about the fact that her breasts aren't natural. She has since gained some increased sensation and that is positive for us both.*
>
> *—Dan*

Issues for Caregivers

Whether family member, partner, or friend, if you're acting as a caregiver to someone who is recovering from mastectomy or reconstruction, it helps to understand the scope of her recovery and know what to expect. Be ready to respond to whatever she needs: cold packs to reduce swelling, a sympathetic ear, or a nice cup of tea. Help her in and out of bed. Be supportive if she has setbacks or complications. Remain calm and patient, particularly if she is used to being independent. She may need help getting into the shower or tub, for example, but if she's strong-minded, she may not like asking for help. Be patient if she is abrupt because she's uncomfortable, worried, or frustrated with her recovery.

If you'll be your mate's primary caregiver, you'll be dealing with two powerful sets of emotions: yours and hers. Being a caregiver can exact its own toll; it's important to balance providing support to her and supporting yourself. Keep the end target in mind: her recovery will one day be over. At times, that may be hard for both of you to keep in perspective. Meanwhile, take care of yourself, because the stress and anxiety you feel can easily undermine your own health. Eat well, get plenty of rest, and allow yourself to get away for short periods to renew your strength and spirit. Ask a relative or close friend to spend the morning with your partner while you head to the office for a few hours, or go for a walk while she has a nap. If you feel stressed, find an outlet for your emotions, especially if you're the strong silent type and it's difficult to talk about your feelings. Speak to a trusted friend, clergyperson, or counselor at your local cancer center. Support groups for partners of cancer survivors, including the National Alliance of Caregiving (www.caregiving.org), can be helpful. Writing about your feelings is also cathartic.

Dos and Don'ts for Friends

As we all know, actions speak louder than words; besides being of practical use, they're a meaningful way to show your feelings, especially if you feel uncomfortable talking about cancer, surgery, or recovery.

Deliver meals. No matter what type of reconstruction your friend has had, she won't be spending time in the kitchen anytime soon. One of the most helpful things you can do is to deliver meals that are easily reheated— and offer to recruit neighbors and friends for meal delivery, if that hasn't already been done. A hearty soup or stew, pizza, pasta, or other main course with a salad and a dessert will be appreciated by the patient and her entire family. It's always nice to throw in extra surprises, like a funny card, cute napkins, a jar of jam, or treats for the family pets.

Babysit. If the patient has children, take them out for an afternoon or stay with them during the day to ensure Mom gets her rest. Invite them over for a sleepover with your kids. Take them to school, soccer practice, play dates, and music lessons.

Run errands. During recovery, everyday errands and chores that keep a home running smoothly will come to a halt unless someone else does them. Ask if you can do grocery shopping (or call while you're at the store to see whether anything is needed). Stocking your friend's kitchen with milk, bread, cereal, eggs, produce, and other grocery essentials the day before she arrives home from the hospital will be a great help. Drop off and pick up dry cleaning, mow the lawn, or walk the dog (maybe even keep the pooch at your house until your friend recovers). Even if your help isn't initially needed, offer again in a few days.

Entertain and amuse. Recovery can be boring between naps. Drop off DVDs, magazines, crossword puzzles, sudoku, and audio books by her favorite author. Send flowers or deliver fresh-cut bouquets from your garden. Perhaps nothing lifts the spirits as much as inspiring words. Your friend will appreciate that you took the time to send e-mails and text messages, and even the most committed technophile enjoys receiving a card in the mail— she can reread your friendly words whenever she needs a little pick-me-up. Don't be afraid to send something humorous; it's good medicine.

A friendly list of don'ts. Unless you've lost your breasts and then had them rebuilt, there's no way to understand the full impact and intense emotions that go along with the experience. Consider the following guidelines to make sure your well-intentioned actions hit the mark.

- Don't resist all contact because you feel awkward or you're nervous about saying the wrong thing. No matter what's going on in your life at the time, your absence or silence will make it seem as though you don't care or aren't interested, and that may strain your relationship. If you're tongue-tied around your friend and don't know what to say, tell her you're sorry she has to go through this experience and that you're there for her when she needs you. Or simply ask, "How are you doing today?" All conversation doesn't need to revolve around reconstruction and recovery. Talk about the weather, what the kids are up to, or what's going on in the neighborhood—the things you would discuss under other circumstances.

- Don't overdo contact, with repeated phone calls or text messages throughout the day. Of course, never show up unannounced—your friend may love a visit, but on some days may not be up to it.
- Don't judge her decisions. It's hard enough to understand all the nuances of mastectomy and reconstruction without having someone second-guess your decisions, especially after the fact. We all make decisions based on our individual priorities and fears. Respect your friend's decisions, even if you disagree with her.
- Don't be squeamish about surgical details your friend would like to share. Breast reconstruction isn't always pretty at first. Try not to grimace or gasp as she explains her procedure in graphic detail, pulls up her shirt to show you her drains, or wants you to see her incisions. Inquire about her surgery, if you're curious, and then respect the extent to which she does or doesn't want to share.
- Don't be afraid to make eye contact. Sometimes people feel so uncomfortable around recovering friends that they're embarrassed to look them in the eye. Even if you feel nervous, maintaining eye contact will show your friend that she has your undivided attention.
- Don't be insensitive to the situation. You probably know of others who have had cancer, and you may know of other women who have had reconstruction, but try to avoid comments such as:

"A co-worker had reconstruction a year ago and she's still in pain."
"You're not considering implants, are you?"
"My aunt had breast cancer, too, and she died."
"I still don't understand why you just didn't have a lumpectomy."
"I can't imagine why you would choose to remove your breasts when you may never develop cancer."

Closing Thoughts

Research is the art of seeing what everyone else has seen, and doing what no one else has done. —ANONYMOUS

Breast reconstruction continues to evolve, as plastic surgeons push the reconstructive envelope. New technologies and techniques refine results, streamline procedures, and shorten recovery. While these innovations benefit women who face mastectomy, science is driving us toward the ultimate goal: a time when mastectomy is archaic and this book will be obsolete. But discovery isn't easy, and the development process isn't quick. Until then, many promising approaches to reconstruction are already in the technology pipeline.

Self-controlled tissue expansion. If a do-it-yourself method of tissue expansion proves successful, the process may become much quicker and far less cumbersome. A new tissue expander that can be inflated with carbon dioxide by the patient at home, at her own convenience, is now undergoing trials. No saline fills are needed, and for most patients, the expander could be fully inflated in just a couple of weeks. It can then be exchanged for a full-sized implant.

Manipulating stem cells to make better use of fat. Liposuction and lipofilling procedures are improving, but the amount of fat that is resorbed by the body still limits the success of these procedures. Your own stem cells may be the key to making fat more viable, so that it will stay where it is needed—in the breast. A new system developed by Cytori Therapeutics, Inc., in Japan uses stem cell–enriched fat to improve lumpectomy defects, and it is producing impressive results. Once fat is liposuctioned, processing isolates and concentrates the stem cells while removing excess blood cells, fluid, and other unwanted substances. The cells are then recombined, and the stem cell–enriched fat is injected into the lumpectomy site. In four to six weeks, the transplanted cells regenerate, filling in the sunken area of the breast. The stem cells don't actually become breast tissue; they encourage the blood supply that the fat cells need to grow and fill out the breast. If the process proves to be safe and effective and gains FDA approval for lumpectomy patients, the obvious next step would be to determine whether it's a potential alternative for women who prefer reconstruction without implants or the ordeal and recovery associated with tissue flap procedures.

A few surgeons have already promoted fat to a starring role in their reconstruction endeavors. The BRAVA Breast Enhancement and Shaping System (www.brava.com) is an unusual alternative to implants and tissue flaps. It uses large, external suction domes that are held in place by a special bra. The device applies gentle, sustained pressure to the chest to expand the skin. The process is based on the concept of induced tension: if you stretch skin and tissue, it grows. This is a reversal of tissue expansion—expanders stretch tissue from the inside, while the BRAVA system stretches it from the outside. Initially, a small application of fat is injected into the chest, so you wake from mastectomy with a small breast mound in place. The BRAVA equipment must then be worn for three to five weeks before microdroplets of your own fat are injected into the breast mound to add volume. The process must be repeated three or four times, a few months apart, to obtain the desired volume. The new breast mound is said to look and feel natural, with full sensation. BRAVA is low-tech and time-intensive, but if it works and does so safely, it would provide a less invasive alternative for mastectomy patients. So far, no controlled, long-term studies of the procedure have been conducted, and the FDA views BRAVA as an unregulated device. Although the procedure may be covered by insurance, the cost of the apparatus isn't.

Tissue engineering. Adult stem cells found in bone marrow and blood are the body's building blocks. They're genetic blank slates, awaiting orders to evolve into bone, lungs, heart, or any kind of tissue the body needs. Researchers believe that stem cells are the key to the body's self-repair—they're learning how to nudge the cells in certain directions to repair cellular defects that cause disease. Stem cell therapy is already being used to replace seriously burned skin and replace cells that are destroyed by the chemotherapy used to treat leukemia and lymphoma. The ultimate goal is to be able to prompt stem cells to regenerate damaged and missing tissue, including limbs and organs. The possibilities are endless, and expectations are high. Stem cells are already showing exciting potential for patients with heart disease, diabetes, arthritis, and other conditions. In the future, it might be possible to generate custom-made hearts, livers, kidneys, and other organs to resolve many life-threatening illnesses. If we can generate new tissue and bone, people with paralyzing spinal cord injuries might walk again. Organ transplants would no longer be needed, and breast reconstruction might be replaced with breast regrowth. As far-fetched as this might seem, the science of tissue engineering is advancing, with practical applications proving successful in the lab and in limited trials.

Will this method regrow breasts? Scientists have already successfully mixed stem cells with a growth factor to "generate" breasts in the lab. Within a year, the stem cells, which grow into a biodegradable breast-shaped scaffolding that is implanted at the mastectomy site, form a new breast.

Gene repair. Scientists are getting closer to unlocking the genetic secrets of many diseases. Sooner or later, they'll discover how to repair defective genes that cause disease. Women diagnosed with breast cancer may undergo gene therapy without needing chemotherapy or radiation. We'll move breast cancer to the list of diseases we no longer need to fear, and mastectomy will no longer be needed. Until then, reconstruction is our best antidote for replacing lost breasts.

Notes

CHAPTER 1. WHY MASTECTOMY?

1. Weiss L. "Early concepts of cancer." *Cancer and Metastasis Reviews* 19, no. 3–4 (2000): 205–17.

2. American Cancer Society. "Surgery for breast cancer—axillary lymph node dissection." www.cancer.org/Cancer/BreastCancer/DetailedGuide/breast-cancer-treating-surgery.

3. Women'sHealth.gov. "Early-stage breast cancer treatment: a patient and doctor dialogue." www.womenshealth.gov/faq/early-stage-breast-cancer.cfm#fm.

4. Giuliano AE, Hunt KK, Ballman KV, et al. "Axillary dissection vs no axillary dissection in women with invasive breast cancer and sentinel node metastasis." *Journal of the American Medical Association* 305, no. 6 (2011): 569–75; Krag DN, Anderson SJ, Jul TB, et al. "Primary outcome results of NSABP B-32, a randomized phase III clinical trial to compare sentinel node resection (SNR) to conventional axillary dissection (AD) in clinically node-negative breast cancer patients." *Journal of Clinical Oncology* 28, no. 18s (suppl., 2010): abstr. LBA505.

5. Van Nes JGH, Seynaeve C, Jones S, et al. "Variations in locoregional therapy in postmenopausal patients with early breast cancer treated in different countries." *British Journal of Surgery* 97, no. 5 (2010): 671–79; Locker GY, Sainsbury JR, and Cuzick J. ATAC Trialists' Group. "Breast surgery in the 'Arimidex, Tamoxifen Alone or in Combination' (ATAC) trial: American women are more likely than women from the United Kingdom to undergo mastectomy." *Cancer* 101, no. 4 (2004): 735–40.

6. Smith GL, Ying X, Ya-Chen TS, et al. "Breast-conserving surgery in older patients with invasive breast cancer: current patterns of treatment across the United States." *Journal of the American College of Surgeons* 209, no. 4 (2009): 425–33.

7. Hawley ST, Griggs JJ, Hamilton AS, et al. "Decision involvement and receipt of mastectomy among racially and ethnically diverse breast cancer patients." *Journal of the National Cancer Institute* 101, no. 19 (2009): 1337–47.

CHAPTER 3. BREAST RECONSTRUCTION BASICS

1. Nedumpara T, Jonker L, and Williams MR. "Impact of immediate breast reconstruction on breast cancer recurrence and survival." *Breast* 20, no. 5 (2011):

437-43; Yi M, Kronowitz SJ, Meric-Bernstam F, et al. "Local, regional, and systemic recurrence rates in patients undergoing skin-sparing mastectomy compared with conventional mastectomy." *Cancer* 117, no. 5 (2011): 916–24.

2. Kulkarni A. "Patterns of use and surgical outcomes of breast reconstruction among obese patients: results from a population-based study." Joint annual scientific meeting of the American Society of Plastic Surgery and the Canadian Society of Aesthetic Plastic Surgery. Presented Oct. 4, 2010 (abstr. 17375).

3. McCarthy CM, Mehrara BJ, Riedel E, et al. "Predicting complications following expander/implant breast reconstruction: an outcomes analysis based on preoperative clinical risk." *Plastic and Reconstructive Surgery* 121, no. 6 (2008): 1886–92.

4. Beahm EK, Walton RL, and Chang DW. "Breast reconstruction in the obese patient." American Society of Plastic Surgeons annual meeting. Presented Oct. 8, 2006; Jandali S, Nelson JA, Sonnad SS, et al. "Breast reconstruction with free tissue transfer from the abdomen in the morbidly obese." *Plastic and Reconstructive Surgery* 127, no. 6 (2011): 2206–13.

5. McCarthy et al. "Predicting complications following expander/implant breast reconstruction."

6. Padubidri AN, Yetman R, Browne E, et al. "Complications of postmastectomy breast reconstructions in smokers, ex-smokers, and nonsmokers." *Plastic and Reconstructive Surgery* 107, no. 2 (2001): 342–49.

7. Alderman AK, Collins ED, Schott A, et al. "The impact of breast reconstruction on the delivery of chemotherapy." *Cancer* 116, no. 7 (2010): 1791–1800; Peled AW, Itakura R, Foster RD, et al. "Impact of chemotherapy on postoperative complications after mastectomy and immediate breast reconstruction." *Archives of Surgery* 145, no. 9 (2010): 880–85.

8. Jhaveri J, Rush SC, Kostroff K, et al. "Clinical outcomes of postmastectomy radiation therapy after immediate breast reconstruction." *International Journal of Radiation Oncology Biology Physics* 72, no. 3 (2008): 859–65.

9. Salgarello M, Visconti G, and Barone-Adesi L. "Fat grafting and breast reconstruction with implant: another option for irradiated breast cancer patients." *Plastic and Reconstructive Surgery* 129, no. 2 (2012): 317–29.

10. Tran NV, Chang DW, Gupta A, et al. "Comparison of immediate and delayed free TRAM flap breast reconstruction in patients receiving postmastectomy radiation therapy." *Plastic and Reconstructive Surgery* 108, no. 1 (2001): 78–82; Rogers NE and Allen RJ. "Radiation effects on breast reconstruction with the deep inferior epigastric perforator flap." *Plastic and Reconstructive Surgery* 109, no. 6 (2002): 1919–26; Spear SL, Ducic I, Low M, et al. "The effect of radiation on pedicled TRAM flap breast reconstruction: outcomes and implications." *Plastic and Reconstructive Surgery* 115, no. 1 (2005): 84–95.

11. Baumann DP, Crosby MA, Selber JC, et al. "Optimal timing of delayed free lower abdominal flap breast reconstruction after postmastectomy radiation therapy." *Plastic and Reconstructive Surgery* 127, no. 3 (2011): 1100–1106.

12. Schechter NR, Strom EA, Perkins GH, et al. "Immediate breast reconstruction can impact postmastectomy irradiation." *American Journal of Clinical Oncology* 28, no. 5 (2005): 485–94.

CHAPTER 4. HOW MASTECTOMY AFFECTS RECONSTRUCTION

1. Golshan M. "Mastectomy," in *Diseases of the Breast*, ed. J. R. Harris et al. (Philadelphia: Lippincott Williams & Wilkins, 2009): 501–6.
2. Shaw WW, Orringer JS, Ko CY, et al. "The spontaneous return of sensibility in breasts reconstructed with autologous tissues." *Plastic and Reconstructive Surgery* 99, no. 2 (1997): 394–99; Nahabedian M. "Nerve regeneration and return of sensation following breast reconstruction with abdominal flaps." www.hopkinsbreast center.org/artemis/200101/feature.html.
3. Stolier AJ and Wang J. "Terminal duct lobular units are scarce in the nipple: implications for prophylactic nipple-sparing mastectomy." *Annals of Surgical Oncology* 15, no. 2 (2008): 438–42; Jensen JA, Orringer JS, and Giuliano AE. "Nipple-sparing mastectomy in 99 patients with a mean follow-up of 5 years." *Annals of Surgical Oncology* 18, no. 6 (2011): 1665–70.
4. Spear SL, Hannan CM, Willey SC, et al. "Nipple-sparing mastectomy." *Plastic and Reconstructive Surgery* 123, no. 6 (2009): 1665–67.
5. Brachtel EF, Rusby JE, Michaelson JS, et al. "Occult nipple involvement in breast cancer: clinicopathologic findings in 316 consecutive mastectomy specimens." *Journal of Clinical Oncology* 27, no. 30 (2009): 4948–54.
6. Petit JY, Veronesi U, Orecchia R, et al. "The nipple sparing mastectomy: a 5-year experience at the European Institute of Oncology of Milan." *Breast Cancer Research* 9 (suppl. 1, 2007): S10.

CHAPTER 5. CONSIDERING PROPHYLACTIC MASTECTOMY

1. Chen S and Parmigiani G. "Meta-analysis of BRCA1 and BRCA2 penetrance." *Journal of Clinical Oncology* 25, no. 11 (2007): 1329–33.
2. Hartmann LC, Schaid DJ, Woods JE, et al. "Efficacy of bilateral prophylactic mastectomy in women with a family history of breast cancer." *New England Journal of Medicine* 340, no. 2 (1999): 77–84; Rebbeck TR, Friebel T, Lynch HT, et al. "Bilateral prophylactic mastectomy reduces breast cancer risk in *BRCA1* and *BRCA2* mutation carriers: the PROSE Study Group." *Journal of Clinical Oncology* 22, no. 6 (2004): 1055–62.
3. Rebbeck TR, Kauff ND, and Domchek SM. "Meta-analysis of risk reduction estimates associated with risk-reducing salpingo-oophorectomy in BRCA1 or BRCA2 mutation carriers." *Journal of the National Cancer Institute* 101, no. 2 (2009): 80–87.
4. Rebbeck TR, Lynch HT, Neuhausen SL, et al. "Prophylactic oophorectomy in

carriers of BRCA1 or BRCA2 mutations." *New England Journal of Medicine* 346, no. 21 (2002): 1616–22.

5. Metcalfe K, Lynch HT, Ghadirian P, et al. "Contralateral breast cancer in BRCA1 and BRCA2 mutation carriers." *Journal of Clinical Oncology* 22, no. 12 (2004): 2328-35; Sorbero ME, Dick AW, Beckjord EB, et al. "Diagnostic breast magnetic resonance imaging and contralateral prophylactic mastectomy." *Annals of Surgical Oncology* 16, no. 6 (2009): 1597–1605.

CHAPTER 6. BREAST IMPLANTS

1. U.S. Food and Drug Administration. "Labeling for approved breast implants 2009." www.fda.gov/medicaldevices/productsandmedicalprocedures/implantsand prosthetics/breastimplants/ucm063743.htm.

2. U.S. Food and Drug Administration. "Anaplastic large cell lymphoma (alcl)." www.fda.gov/medicaldevices/productsandmedicalprocedures/implantsandprosthe tics/breastimplants/ucm239995.htm.

3. Suber J, Malafa M, Smith P, et al. "Prosthetic breast reconstruction after implant-sparing mastectomy in patients with submuscular implants." *Annals of Plastic Surgery* 66, no. 5 (2011): 546–50; Spear SL, Clemens MW, and Dayan JH. "Considerations of previous augmentation in subsequent breast reconstruction." *Aesthetic Surgery Journal* 28, no. 3 (2008): 285–93.

4. Salzberg CA, Ashikari AY, Koch RM, et al. "An 8-year experience of direct-to-implant immediate breast reconstruction using human acellular dermal matrix (Alloderm)." *Plastic and Reconstructive Surgery* 127, no. 2 (2011): 514–24.

5. Hölmich LR, Kjøller K, Vejborg I, et al. "Prevalence of silicone breast implant rupture among Danish women." *Plastic and Reconstructive Surg*ery 108, no. 4 (2001): 848-58; Hölmich LR, Vejborg IM, Conrad C, et al. "Untreated silicone breast implant rupture." *Plastic and Reconstructive Surg*ery 114, no. 1 (2004): 204–14.

CHAPTER 7. THE EXPANDER EXPERIENCE

1. Layeeque R, Hochberg J, Siegel E, et al. "Botulinum toxin infiltration for pain control after mastectomy and expander reconstruction." *Annals of Surgery* 240, no. 4 (2004): 608–14; Wong WW, Gabriel A, Maxwell GP, et al. "The efficacy of botulinum toxin in post mastectomy expansion." *Plastic and Reconstructive Surgery* 125, no. 6 (2010): 28.

CHAPTER 8. TUMMY TUCK FLAPS

1. Seidenstuecker K, Munder B, Mahajan AL, et al. "Morbidity of microsurgical breast reconstruction in patients with comorbid conditions." *Plastic and Reconstructive Surgery* 127, no. 3 (2011): 1086–92.

2. DellaCroce FJ, Sullivan SK, and Trahan C. "Stacked deep inferior epigastric perforator flap breast reconstruction: a review of 110 flaps in 55 cases over 3 years." *Plastic and Reconstructive Surgery* 127, no. 3 (2011): 1093–99.

CHAPTER 9. OTHER FLAP METHODS

1. Disa JJ, McCarthy CM, Mehrara BJ, et al. "Immediate latissimus dorsi/prosthetic breast reconstruction following salvage mastectomy after failed lumpectomy/irradiation." *Plastic and Reconstructive Surgery* 121, no. 4 (2008): 159e–64e; Spear SL, Boehmler JH, Taylor NS, et al. "The role of the latissimus dorsi flap in reconstruction of the irradiated breast." *Plastic and Reconstructive Surgery* 119, no. 1 (2007): 1–9.

2. Saint-Cyr M, Nagarkar P, Schaverien M, et al. "The pedicled descending branch muscle-sparing latissimus dorsi flap for breast reconstruction." *Plastic and Reconstructive Surgery* 123, no. 1 (2009): 13–24.

3. DellaCroce FJ and Sullivan SK. "Application and refinement of the superior gluteal artery perforator free flap for bilateral simultaneous breast reconstruction." *Plastic and Reconstructive Surgery* 116, no. 1 (2005): 97–103.

4. Saint-Cyr M, Shirvani A, and Wong C. "The transverse upper gracilis flap for breast reconstruction following liposuction of the thigh." *Microsurgery* 30, no. 8 (2010): 636–38.

CHAPTER 11. FINAL TOUCHES: CREATING YOUR NIPPLE AND AREOLA

1. McCarthy CM, VanLaeken N, Lennox P, et al. "The efficacy of Artecoll injections for the augmentation of nipple projection in breast reconstruction." *Eplasty* 10 (2010): e7.

CHAPTER 15. DEALING WITH PROBLEMS

1. Khansa I, Colakoglu S, Curtis MS, et al. "Postmastectomy breast reconstruction after previous lumpectomy and radiation therapy: analysis of complications and satisfaction." *Annals of Plastic Surgery* 66, no. 5 (2011): 444–51.

2. Macdonald L, Bruce J, Scott NW, et al. "Long-term follow-up of breast cancer survivors with post-mastectomy pain syndrome." *British Journal of Cancer* 92, no. 2 (2005): 225–30; Gärtner R, Jensen MB, Nielsen J, et al. "Prevalence of and factors associated with persistent pain following breast cancer surgery." *Journal of the American Medical Association* 302, no 18 (2009): 1985–92; Loftus LS and Laronga C. "Evaluating patients with chronic pain after breast cancer surgery: the search for relief." *Journal of the American Medical Association* 302, no. 18 (2009): 2034–35.

3. Schmitz KH, Ahmed RL, Troxel A, et al. "Weight lifting in women with

breast cancer–related lymphedema." *New England Journal of Medicine* 361, no. 7 (2009): 664–73.

4. Khan S. "Axillary reverse mapping to prevent lymphedema after breast cancer surgery: defining the limits of the concept." *Journal of Clinical Oncology* 27, no. 33 (2009): 5494–96.

5. Becker C, Assouad J, Riquet M, et al. "Postmastectomy lymphedema: long-term results following microsurgical lymph node transplantation." *Annals of Surgery* 243, no 3 (2006): 313–15.

6. Petit JY, Botteri E, Lohsiriwat V, et al. "Locoregional recurrence risk after lipofilling in breast cancer patients." *Annals of Oncology* 223, no. 3 (2012): 802–3.

CHAPTER 18. PAYING FOR YOUR RECONSTRUCTION

1. Alderman AK, Dunya A, Streu R, et al. "Patterns and correlates of postmastectomy breast reconstruction by U.S. plastic surgeons: results from a national survey." *Plastic and Reconstructive Surgery* 127, no. 5 (2011): 1796–1803.

Glossary

Acellular dermal matrix (ADM) Donor skin that has been stripped of its cellular material and sterilized, and then is used to replace missing tissue.

Adjuvant therapy Treatment given after surgery.

Anterolateral perforator flap A flap of skin and fat taken from the front of the thigh that is used to recreate a breast.

Areola The circle of darkened skin around the nipple.

Areola-sparing mastectomy A procedure that removes most of the breast tissue and nipple but preserves the breast skin and areola.

Asymmetry Uneven size, shape, or position of one breast relative to the other.

Attached flap A flap of skin, fat, and muscle that remains connected to its original blood supply and is tunneled under the skin from the donor site to the chest to recreate a new breast; also called pedicled flap.

Attached TRAM flap A flap of abdominal skin, fat, and muscle that remains connected to its original blood supply and is tunneled under the skin to the chest to recreate a new breast; also called pedicled TRAM.

Augmentation mammoplasty Plastic surgery to increase breast size.

Autologous reconstruction A reconstruction that is accomplished with a person's own tissue.

Axillary node dissection Surgical removal of underarm lymph nodes to determine whether cancer has spread beyond the breast.

Axillary reverse mapping A procedure to evaluate patterns of fluid drainage from the breast to the lymph node system.

Benign Non-cancerous.

Bilateral mastectomy Surgical removal of both breasts.

Bilateral reconstruction Recreation of both breasts after mastectomy.

Bilateral salpingo-oophorectomy (BSO) Surgery to remove the ovaries.

Biopsy Removal and examination of sample cells, fluid, or tissue.

BRCA1 and BRCA2 (BReast CAncer genes 1 and 2) Genes that, when mutated, significantly increase the risk of developing breast and ovarian cancers.

Breast augmentation Surgery to enlarge a breast with an implant.

Breast cancer Uncontrolled growth of abnormal breast cells.

Breast implant An artificial device that replaces missing breast tissue after mastectomy.

Breast lift (mastopexy) Surgery to reposition a breast higher on the chest.

Breast mound A reconstructed breast without a nipple or areola.

Breast reconstruction Surgery that uses an implant or a patient's own tissue to restore breast shape and volume after mastectomy.

Breast reduction (reduction mammoplasty) Surgery to reduce the size of the breast.

Capsular contracture Tightening of the scar capsule surrounding an implant.

Capsulectomy Surgery to remove hard scar tissue around an implant.

Capsulotomy A procedure that attempts to break the capsule of scar tissue surrounding an implant by compressing it.

Chemotherapy Drug treatment used to destroy cancer cells.

Clinical trial A scientific study using human subjects, conducted to determine whether a drug or procedure is safe and effective.

Cohesive gel A type of viscous silicone implant filling.

Collagen Connective tissue protein produced by the body.

Computed tomography (CT or CAT) scan An x-ray that produces sectional images of the body.

Contralateral mastectomy Removal of the opposite, healthy breast.

Co-payment (co-pay) A fixed amount, predetermined by your health insurance policy, that you are required to pay before you receive medical services or prescriptions.

Debride Remove unhealthy tissue.

Deductible The amount you must pay out-of-pocket for medical expenses or prescriptions before your health insurance begins paying.

Deep inferior epigastric perforator (DIEP) flap A muscle-preserving flap of abdominal fat and skin that is used to recreate a breast.

Delay procedure A minor procedure, performed before abdominal flap reconstruction, that divides blood vessels in the lower abdomen to increase blood supply to blood vessels in the upper abdomen.

Delayed-immediate reconstruction Placement of a tissue expander to preserve breast shape and facilitate reconstruction for individuals who may require post-mastectomy radiation.

Delayed reconstruction Surgery to recreate a breast after recovery from mastectomy.

Delayed wound healing A wound that is slow to heal.

Dermis The underlying tissue that supports the skin.

Direct-to-implant reconstruction Single-step reconstruction that places a full-sized implant immediately after nipple-sparing mastectomy; also called non-expansive, one-step, or single-stage implant reconstruction.

Dog ears Puckered ends of a scar.

Donor site Any location on the body where tissue is borrowed to recreate a breast.

Doppler An instrument that evaluates blood flow.

Duct The part of the breast that delivers milk to the nipple.

Ductal carcinoma in situ (DCIS) Non-invasive cancer that begins in the breast ducts.

Endoscopic latissimus dorsi reconstruction A reconstructive procedure that transfers the back muscle to the breast site entirely through the mastectomy incision or a small incision under the arm.

Epidermis The outer layer of skin.

Exchange surgery A secondary reconstructive operation to replace a tissue expander with an implant.

Extended DIEP flap Skin and fat from the abdomen and hip that are combined to recreate a breast.

Extended latissimus dorsi flap A flap that uses the back muscle and the surrounding fat to create a new breast.

Extrusion A condition in which an implant pokes through the skin.

Fascia The fibrous tissue covering the muscles.

Fat grafting Transferring liposuctioned body fat to the reconstructed breast to improve small cosmetic imperfections; also called lipofilling.

Flap An island of skin, fat, tissue, and sometimes muscle that is moved from one location on the body to another to replace missing tissue.

Free flap Tissue that is transferred, along with its blood supply and a small portion of muscle, from one location on the body to another.

Free TRAM flap Abdominal fat, skin, and a small portion of muscle used to recreate a breast.

Galactorrhea A spontaneous milky discharge from the breast that may occur after breast augmentation.

Genetic Related to or influenced by genes.

Genetic counselor A health professional who is trained to interpret patterns in a family's medical history and estimate an individual's risk for disease.

Genetic mutation A change in a gene that may cause cancer.

Genetic testing Laboratory examination of a person's blood sample to determine whether she has a genetic mutation.

Gluteal artery perforator (GAP) flap Skin and fat taken from the buttocks to recreate a breast.

Granuloma A small area of inflamed tissue that sometimes develops around sutures.

Hematoma A collection of blood outside the blood vessels.

Hereditary breast cancer A cancer caused by a gene mutation passed from one generation to another.

Hernia The protrusion of an organ through a weakened muscle.

Hypertrophic scar A scar that rises above the level of the surrounding skin and may be painful or tender.

Immediate reconstruction Surgery to recreate a breast, directly following a mastectomy and while the patient is still sedated.

Inferior gluteal artery perforator (IGAP) flap Skin and fat taken from the lower buttock to recreate a breast.

Infiltrating ductal carcinoma (IDC) The most common form of breast cancer, which develops in the breast ducts; also called invasive ductal carcinoma.

Inframammary fold The crease under the breast.

In-network A group of doctors, hospitals, or other medical providers that are contracted with a particular health insurance company to accept predetermined fees for services.

Intercostal artery perforator (ICAP) flap A small amount of underarm tissue that can be used to fill out lumpectomy defects.

Intercostobrachial neuralgia (ICN) Pain caused by severing of the intercostobrachial nerve.

Invasive breast cancer Cancer that can spread beyond the breast.

Keloid A thick scar that spreads into the skin around an incision.

Lateral transverse thigh flap A flap of skin and fat from the outer thigh that is used to recreate a breast; also called Reubens flap.

Latissimus dorsi (lat) flap A flap of skin, fat, and muscle from the back that is tunneled under the skin to the chest to recreate a breast.

Lobe The part of the breast that produces milk; also called lobule.

Lumbar artery perforator (LAP) flap Skin and fat from the upper hip and waist used to recreate a breast.

Lumpectomy Surgery to remove a breast tumor and a small amount of surrounding tissue.

Lymph nodes Small glands that filter impurities in the body.

Lymph system A network of small glands, connected by lymphatic vessels, that filter impurities in the body.

Lymphedema Swelling in the arm or extremities caused by excess fluid after lymph nodes are removed or the breast is irradiated.

Magnetic resonance imaging (MRI) A type of scan that uses magnets instead of radiation to produce images of the body's interior or detect ruptured breast implants.

Malignant Cancerous.

Malposition In the wrong position.

Mammogram An x-ray used to identify breast tissue abnormalities, including cancer.

Mammoplasty (augmentation) Plastic surgery to increase breast size.

Mastectomy Surgical removal of the breast.

Mastopexy (breast lift) Surgery to reposition a breast higher on the chest.

Metastasis The spread of cancer beyond its original location.

Microsurgeon A medical professional trained to perform intricate operations with special precision instruments.

Microsurgery Delicate surgery that requires special training and equipment to re-connect blood vessels.

Modified radical mastectomy Removal of breast tissue, skin, some or all of the un-derarm lymph nodes, and the lining over the chest muscle.

Muscle-sparing latissimus dorsi flap Back skin, fat, and some muscle used to re-create a breast.

Muscle-sparing TRAM flap Abdominal skin, fat, and a postage-stamp size portion of muscle used to recreate a breast.

Necrosis Tissue or cell death.

Neoadjuvant therapy Treatment given before surgery.

Nipple reconstruction A surgical procedure that recreates new nipples after mastectomy.

Nipple sharing Using part of a woman's healthy nipple to create a new nipple on the opposite reconstructed breast.

Nipple-sparing mastectomy (NSM) A procedure that removes the breast tissue but preserves most breast skin, nipple, and areola.

Non-invasive breast cancer Cancer that doesn't spread beyond the breast.

Oncologist A physician who specializes in the treatment of cancer.

Out-of-network Doctors, hospitals, and other medical providers that aren't con-tracted with a particular health insurance company to accept predetermined fees for services.

Out-of-pocket cost The total amount you pay for medical services not covered by your health insurance.

Outpatient procedure A procedure that doesn't require an overnight hospital stay.

Pathologist A physician who determines whether cancerous cells are present in tis-sue samples.

Pectoralis muscles Muscles under the breast; includes the pectoralis major and pectoralis minor muscles.

Pedicled flap A flap of skin, fat, and muscle that remains connected to its original blood supply and is tunneled under the skin from the donor site to the chest to recreate a new breast; also called attached flap.

Perforator flap A muscle-preserving flap of fat and skin that is used to recreate a breast.

Perforator vessels Small arteries that run throughout muscle.

Periareolar Around the areola.

Periumbilical perforator (PUP) flap A type of muscle-sparing abdominal flap used to recreate a breast.

Phantom sensation A perceived feeling from a missing body part.

Plastic surgeon A medical professional who specializes in cosmetic or reconstructive surgery.

Plastic surgery An operation performed to improve appearance.

Post-mastectomy pain syndrome Pain that persists after recovery from mastectomy.

Previvor Someone who has an inherited predisposition to cancer, but cancer hasn't been diagnosed.

Profunda artery perforator (PAP) flap A flap of skin and fat from the upper thigh below the buttock that is used to recreate a breast.

Prophylactic bilateral mastectomy (PBM) Surgical removal of both breasts to reduce the risk of developing breast cancer.

Prosthesis A breast form worn in clothing to give the appearance of natural breasts.

Pulse oximeter A device that measures the level of oxygen in blood.

Quadrantectomy A type of lumpectomy that removes about one-fourth of the tissue in a breast.

Radiation therapy Treatment with high-energy waves to destroy cancer cells and prevent recurrence.

Radical mastectomy Rarely performed procedure in which the entire breast, nipple, areola, chest muscles, and underarm lymph nodes are removed.

Re-excision A surgical technique that reopens a wound to remove cancerous, infected, or dead tissue.

Resorb To absorb again, as when the body reassimilates blood or fluid after surgery.

Reubens flap A flap of skin and fat from the outer thigh that is used to recreate a breast; also called lateral transverse thigh flap.

Revision surgery A surgical procedure to improve the results of an earlier operation.

Rupture A breach in the shell of an implant.

Saline A sterile saltwater solution that is used to fill expanders and some breast implants.

Scar A permanent change in the texture of the skin that grows over a wound.

Scar revision Surgery to improve the appearance of a scar.

Sentinel node biopsy A minimally invasive method of sampling lymph nodes to determine whether cancer has spread beyond the breast; also called sentinel node dissection or sentinel node mapping.

Seroma A collection of fluid under the skin.

Silent rupture An undetected leak in a silicone implant.

Silicone A synthetic gel that is used to fill some implants.

Skin graft Healthy skin that is transferred from one part of the body to another to replace damaged or missing skin.

Skin-sparing mastectomy A procedure that removes breast tissue, including the nipple and areola, but preserves most of the breast skin to facilitate immediate reconstruction.

Spirometer A device that expands the lungs and strengthens breathing after surgery.

Stacked DIEP A combination of two abdominal flaps of fat and skin to recreate a single breast; also called double DIEP.

Subcutaneous mastectomy An outdated procedure that deliberately left breast tissue behind during breast cancer surgery to preserve a patient's nipple and areola.

Superficial inferior epigastric artery (SIEA) flap A muscle-preserving flap of abdominal fat and skin used to recreate a breast.

Superior gluteal artery perforator (SGAP) flap Skin and fat taken from the upper buttock to rebuild a breast.

Surgical drain A plastic bulb that collects fluids at the incision site after surgery.

Surgical oncologist A physician who specializes in surgery to treat cancer.

Survivor Someone who has been successfully treated for cancer.

Symmastia Breasts that join together in the center of the chest.

Symmetry Breasts that appear to be of equal proportion, size, and shape.

Tattoo Pigment added beneath the skin.

Thoracodorsal artery perforator (TAP or TDAP) flap A muscle-sparing flap of back tissue.

Tissue expander A temporary saline implant used to gradually stretch skin and muscle to make room for a full-sized implant.

Tissue flap An island of skin, fat, tissue, and sometimes muscle that is moved from one location on the body to another to replace missing tissue.

Total mastectomy Removal of the breast tissue, skin, and nipple to prevent or treat cancer; also called simple mastectomy.

Transumbilical breast augmentation (TUBA) Breast augmentation performed entirely through an incision around the belly button.

Transverse rectus abdominis myocutaneous (TRAM) flap Skin, fat, and some or all of the abdominal muscle used to reconstruct a breast.

Transverse upper gracilis (TUG) flap Skin, fat, and muscle taken from the upper thigh to recreate a breast.

Transverse upper thigh (TUT) flap Skin and fat taken from the upper thigh to recreate a breast.

Unilateral mastectomy Removal of one breast.

Unilateral reconstruction Recreation of one breast after mastectomy.

Vascularized lymph node transfer A surgical procedure to replace previously removed lymph nodes with other healthy nodes.

The Women's Health and Cancer Rights Act (WHCRA) Legislation (1998) requiring health insurance companies that pay for mastectomy to also pay for prostheses and reconstruction surgery.

Resources

BREAST CANCER

American Cancer Society (www.cancer.org)
Breast Cancer Network of Strength (www.y-me.org)
BreastCancer.org (www.breastcancer.org)
Mothers Supporting Daughters with Breast Cancer (http://mothersdaughters.org)
National Cancer Institute (www.cancer.gov)
Susan G. Komen Breast Cancer Foundation (www.komen.org)
Young Survival Coalition (www.youngsurvival.org)
Crazy Sexy Cancer Survivor and *Crazy Sexy Cancer Tips* by Kris Carr

BREAST CANCER GENETICS AND RISK

Facing Our Risk of Cancer Empowered (www.facingourrisk.org)
Informed Medical Decisions (www.informeddna.com)
National Society of Genetic Counselors (www.nsgc.org)
Confronting Hereditary Breast and Ovarian Cancer by Sue Friedman, DVM,
    Rebecca Sutphen, MD, and Kathy Steligo
In the Family (DVD), Kartemquin Films

COPING

The Cancer Club (www.cancerclub.com)
Kids Konnected (www.kidskonnected.org)
Laughter Yoga (www.laughteryoga.org)
National Alliance of Caregivers (www.caregiving.org)
Breast Cancer Husband by Marc Silver
Intimacy after Breast Cancer: Dealing with Your Body, Relationships, and Sex
    by Gina M. Maisano
Prepare for Surgery, Heal Faster (www.healfaster.com)
Why I Wore Lipstick to My Mastectomy by Geralyn Lucas

INSURANCE AND PAYMENT ISSUES

Cancer Care (www.cancercare.org)
CareCredit (www.carecredit.com)
Insurance Information Institute (www.iii.org)
My Hope Chest (www.myhopechest.org)
National Insurance Consumer Helpline (www.consumerservicesguide.org)
Patient Advocate Foundation (www.patientadvocate.org)
The United Breast Cancer Foundation (www.ubcf.info)
The Women's Health and Cancer Rights Act (http://www.dol.gov/ebsa/publications
   /whcra.html)

MASTECTOMY

Amoena (www.amoena.com)
Breast Free (www.breastfree.org)
The Breast Preservation Foundation (www.breastpreservationfoundation.org)
EmbracingMastectomy.com (www.embracingmastectomy.com)
Flattops (http://flattops.webs.com)
Nearly Me (www.nearlyme.org)
Reach to Recovery (www.cancer.org/treatment/supportprogramsservices/
   reach-to-recovery)
Rub-on Nipples (www.tattooednipples.com)
TLC (www.tlcdirect.org)

RECONSTRUCTION

Allergan (www.natrelle.com)
American Society of Plastic Surgeons (www.plasticsurgery.org)
BreastImplantSafety.org (www.breastimplantsafety.org)
The Cancer Survivors Network (http://csn.cancer.org/forum)
Food and Drug Administration (www.fda.gov; search for "breast implants")
Johns Hopkins Medicine (www.hopkinsbreastcenter.org/services/ask_expert)
Mentor (www.yourbreastoptions.com)
Myself: Together Again (www.myselftogetheragain.org)

RECOVERY

Annie & Isabel hospital gowns (www.annieandisabel.com)

The Lance Armstrong Foundation (www.livestrong.com/
   article/28314-post-mastectomy-exercises)

Marsupial (www.turnerhealth.com)

National Lymphedema Network (www.lymphnet.org)

Essential Exercises for Breast Cancer Survivors by Amy Halverstadt and Andrea
   Leonard

Exercises after Breast Surgery (www.cancer.org)

Yoga and the Gentle Art of Healing: A Journey of Recovery after Breast Cancer
   (www.yogajoyofdelmar.com)

Index

ABOUT THE AUTHOR

Kathy Steligo is a health writer and co-author of *Confronting Hereditary Breast and Ovarian Cancer.* Since 2002, she has counseled women about their post-mastectomy options, explaining techniques, clarifying issues, and answering questions so that women understand their choices. She also conducts breast reconstruction seminars and provides writing workshops for women who are dealing with cancer issues. A two-time breast cancer survivor, Kathy has twice had breast reconstruction.